Oh's

오지은의 메디컬 영어회화

.General Hospital

part.3

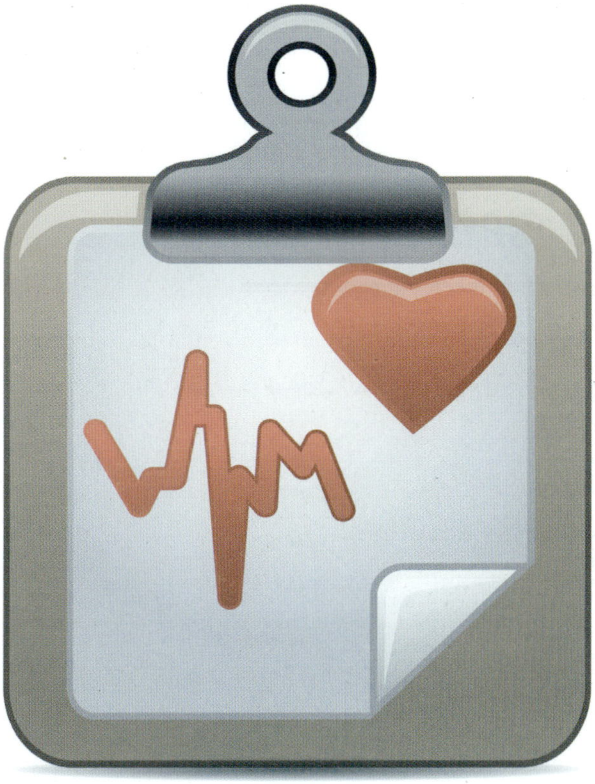

오지은의 메디컬 영어회화 part 3

2011년 10월 1일 초판인쇄
2011년 10월 10일 초판발행

지은이 / 오지은
펴낸이 / 이상태
펴낸곳 / 청구문화사
120-831 서울특별시 서대문구 연희1동 436-1
전 화 / 02) 332-0541(代)
팩 스 / 02) 337-9577
등 록 / 1990년 11월 2일 제9-247호

ISBN 978-89-5616-471-7 93510

정가 35,000원

The Story of 오지은의 메디컬 영어회화. General Hospital

오지은의 메디컬 영어회화. General Hospital은 2009년 4월부터 시작하여 2011년 1월 7일에 완성한 저의 첫 번째 메디컬 영어회화책인 종합병원 편입니다.

이 책은 두 가지의 숙제를 풀고 싶은 마음에서 집필하였습니다. 첫 번째 숙제는, 의료 통역이란 난제의 답을 찾는 실마리가 되어 의료관광이라는 현장에서 선구자의 역할을 하시는 의료 통역사/의료통역 코디네이터 분들에게 영어권 환자분들의 의료 및 생활 문화와 현지의 살아있는 영어를 알려드리고 싶었습니다. "영어권 환자들은 어디에서 왔는가?" 란 질문에 대한 답을 아실 때 의료통역은 한결 더 수월해지실 것이라 생각됩니다. 두 번째 숙제는 해외에 특히 미국으로 진출하시려는 의료종사자분 들의 "우리는 어디로 가는가?"에 대한 답을 드리고 싶었습니다. 저는 미국 University of Utah에서 세포병리학을 전공했고 세포병리사로 미국의 병리 연구 산업기관인 ARUP Laboratories, Inc와 유타주의 지역 병원인 Ogdon Regional Hospital에서 근무를 하였습니다. 아는 만큼 보인다는 격언이 있듯이 십여 년이 넘는 제 미국생활의 경험을 미국 의료 시장으로 진출을 준비하시고 계시는 분들께 알려드리고 싶었습니다. 미국에 도착 후 가장 먼저 만들어야 하는 Social Security Card를 Chapter 1에 실은 이유도 여기에 있습니다. 언어는 문화입니다. 그리고 세 번째의 숙제를 추가하자면 아직 재학중인 보건계열 학생 여러분들이 졸업 전에 이 책을 공부하고 졸업 후 내딛는 사회의 첫 발에 도움이 되었으면 하는 바람입니다. "영어는 권력이다" 라는 항간에 회자되는 말에 저는 영어는 "많은 문을 열어 줄 수 있는 열쇠이다"를 첨가하고 싶습니다. 끝으로 감사의 말을 전하고 싶습니다. 현재 의료 현장에 근무하시며 각자의 꿈을 이루기 위해 향학열을 불태우시는 소중한 오지은의 메디컬 영어회화 1

기생인, 김수민, 최현경, 허선희, 장수경간호사님과 특히 제게 한국의료문화에 대해 많은 조언을 주는 나의 동지인 순천향대학병원의 송선주 간호사님께 큰 감사를 드립니다. 또한 이비인후과 박상철 의사선생님, 조현재 치과 의사선생님, 수원 아주 대학교병원의 약사님, 서울아산병원의 김주연 간호사님, 박소영 의료통역사님, 박안례 의료통역사님, 최영주 아로마테라피 연구소장님 이가영 약사님 외에 제 강의를 수강하신 모든 분들의 소중한 자문으로 이 책이 세상 밖에 나올 수 있었습니다. 현장의 소리를 담은 책이 되고 싶은 제 꿈을 그 분들이 가능하게 해 주셨습니다. 그리고 가장 핵심 과제였던 이 책이 지향하는 방향을 설정하는데 사려 깊은 조언을 주신 정동혁 병원경영 컨설턴트님께 깊은 감사와 고마움을 전합니다. 또한 메디컬 외국어회화를 전공과목으로 한국대학교에 처음 개설하신 김천대학교 의료경영학과의 박지원교수님과 청구문화사 이상태 사장님을 비롯한 직원들의 노고에 감사를 드립니다.

이 책의 제목, 표지 디자인 및 녹음파일 등 다양한 콘텐츠를 이용하실 수 있는 www.ohgieun.com 홈페이지는 B&M Company의 작품입니다. 그들은 천재입니다. 그들에게 무한한 감사의 마음을 전합니다.

Introduction

Part 3는 외국인 환자분들의 진료 후 발생 가능한 혈액검사, 소변 검사, 방사선 검사 및 체온, 맥박, 혈압, 호흡수를 측정하는 활력징후로 구성하였습니다.

일곱 번째 장인 혈액검사및 소변검사에서는 외국인 환자분들이 받으시는 일반적인 혈액검사와 공복 시 행해지는 혈액검사의 소개와 소변 검사 중 일반 소변검사와 24시간 소변검사에 관련된 주요어휘, 주요구문, 및 각 상황에 맞는 대화로 구성하였습니다.

여덟 번째 장은 방사선 검사입니다. 방사선 검사는 외국인 환자의 흉부 방사선 촬영과 복부방사선 촬영에 관련된 진행 절차를 주요어휘, 주요구문, 독해구문 및 다양한 연습문제로 소개하였습니다.

아홉 번째 장은 활력징후입니다. 체온, 맥박, 혈압, 호흡수의 측정 및 신체 계측과 관련된 주요어휘, 주요구문, 독해구문 및 다양한 연습문제로 구성 되어 있습니다.

Part 3의 혈액검사 및 소변검사, 방사선 검사와 활력징후는 수술 편으로 이어집니다. Part 4는 **Chapter 10: 마취**, **Chapter 11: 수술 전 과정** 및 **Chapter 12: 수술 후 관리**로 구성하였습니다. **Part 4**에서 뵙겠습니다.

Special Thanks

Without the Karls, I couldn't finish my first book.

I really appreciate all of your help and support.

Synghoon Karl

Ji-Won Karl

Min-Kyu Karl

Love,

From the bottom of my heart

Part 3

Contents

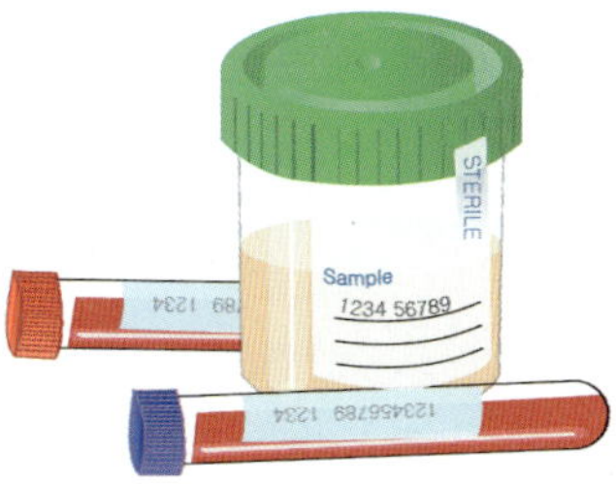

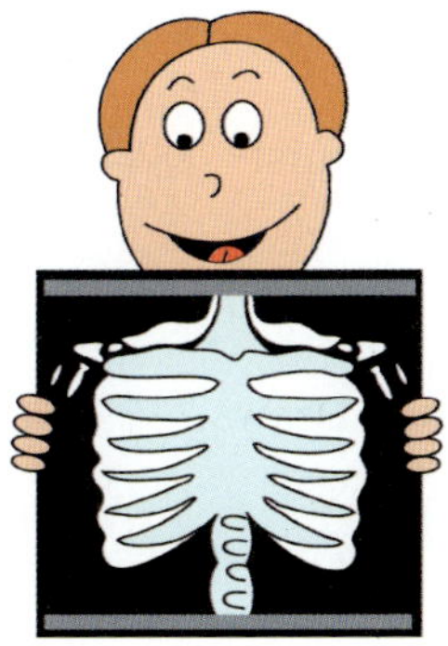

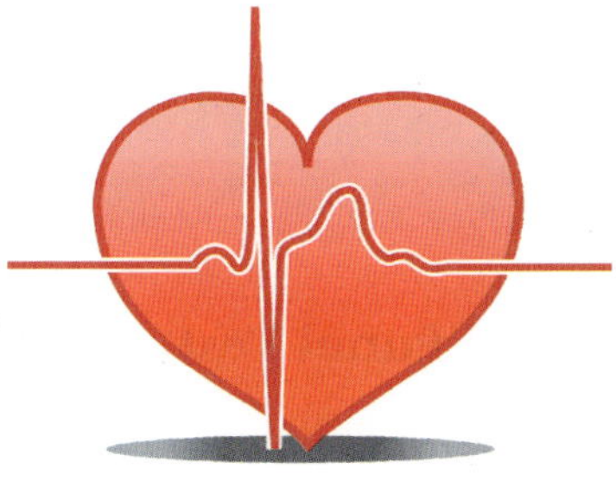

Chapter 7. Blood Work/Urinalysis

1. Blood Work/Blood Test, 혈액검사

2. Cholesterol Test/Lipid Panel Test, 콜레스테롤검사/지질검사

9. Random Urinalysis, 일반 소변 검사

10. 24-hour Urinalysis, 24시간 소변검사

11. FAQ for the Lab Test, 검사에 관련된 자주하는 질문

12. 해석 및 정답

Chapter 8. X-ray Examination

1. X-ray Examination, 방사선 검사

2. Body Temperature (BT), 체온

3. Pulse Rate (PR), 맥박

4. Blood Pressure (BP), 혈압

Chapter 7

Blood Work/Urinalysis

혈액검사 및 소변검사

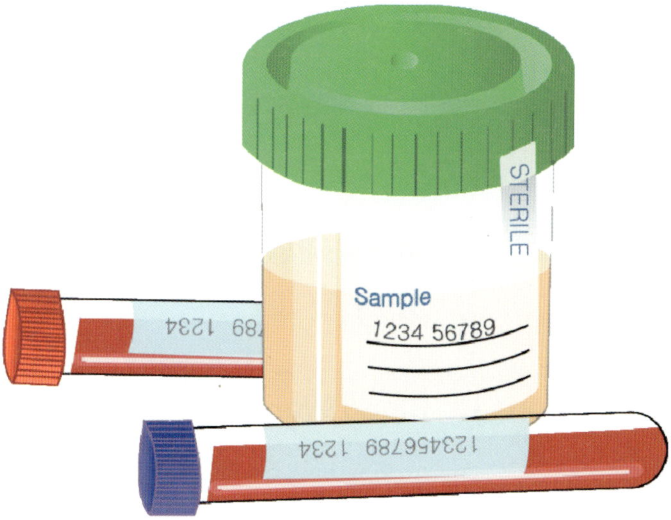

1. Blood Work/Blood Test

혈액검사

· **Key Words, 주요어휘**

■ QUIZ: 내 단어장 점검하기

■ Drill: Word Search Puzzle, 연습문제: 어휘퍼즐

· **Reading Material: My Blood Work!, 독해구문: 나의 혈액검사**

■ Words, 어휘

· **Code Breaker's Corner: 로리와 함께하는 미국 문화 엿보기**

■ What is a Phlebotomist? 채혈사란?

■ Words, 어휘

· **Facts about Blood Draws, 채혈에 관하여**

■ Words, 어휘

· **Key Expressions for Blood Work, 혈액검사관련 주요구문**

■ Words, 어휘

■ Drill, 연습문제

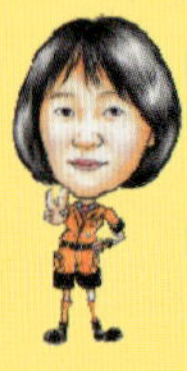

이 책의 녹음 파일은 www.ohgieun.com 에서

무료다운로드 하실 수 있습니다

Key Words

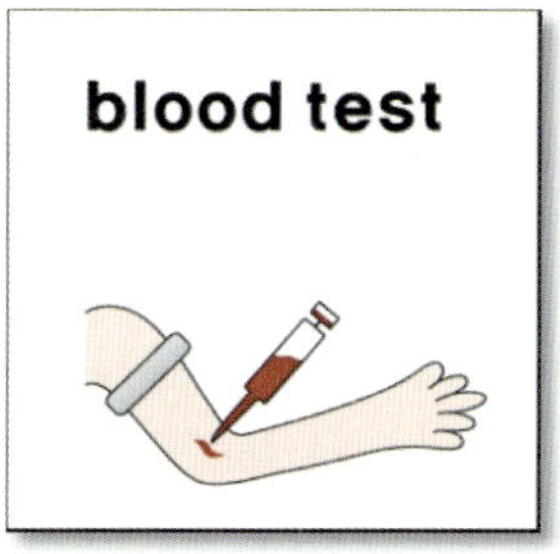

A Blood test/A Blood work: 혈액검사

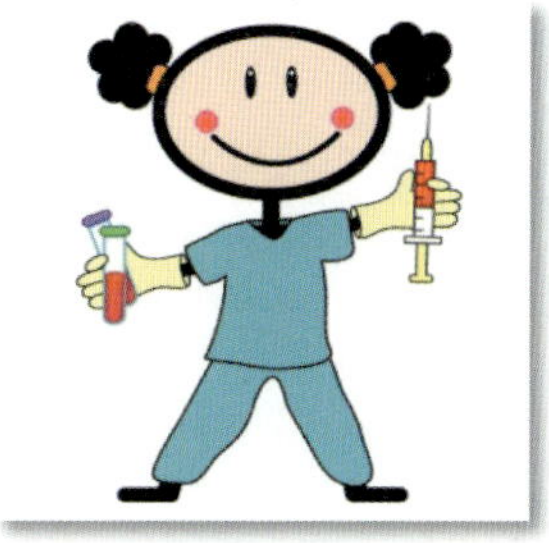

Phlebotomist (A professional who draws blood): 채혈사

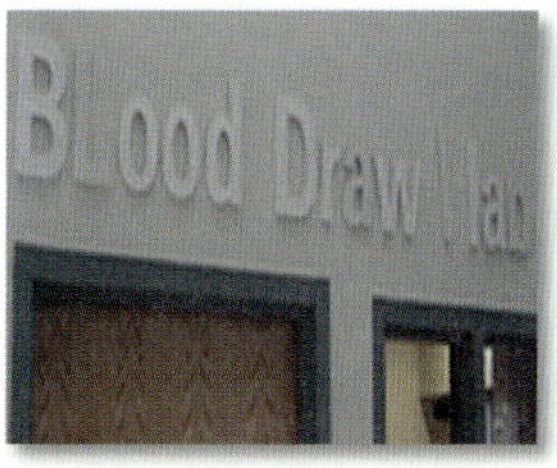

Blood drawing room: 채혈실

Blood lab: 혈액검사실

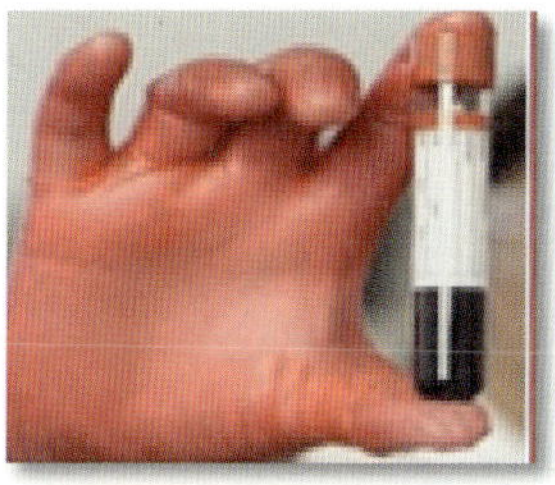

**Blood test vial/Blood tube/
Blood collection tube:**
혈액검체 용기

Key Words

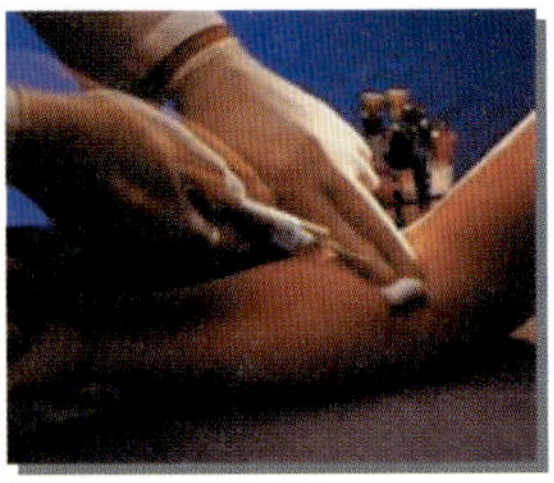

Venipuncture blood test: 정맥채혈

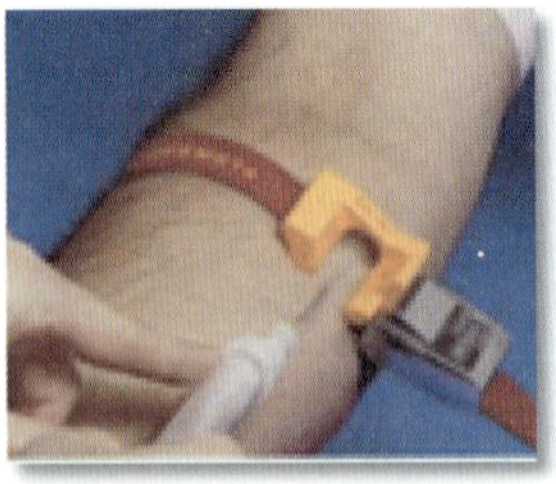

Tourniquet/Rubber cord:
토니켓/압박고무줄

A tourniquet is placed on your arm to make your veins more noticeable to the technician.

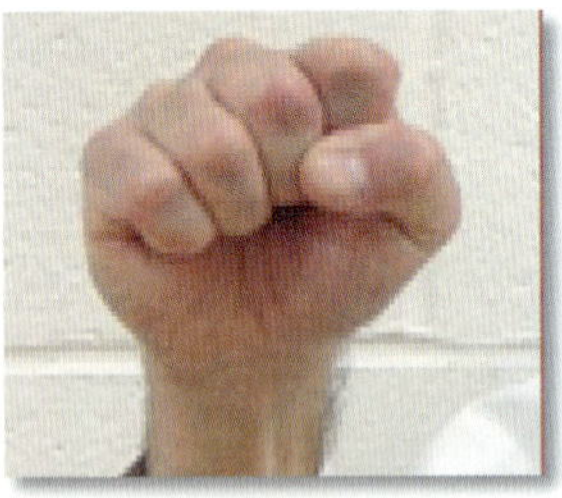

Make a fist: 주먹을 쥐다

Make a tight fist: 주먹을 꽉 쥐다

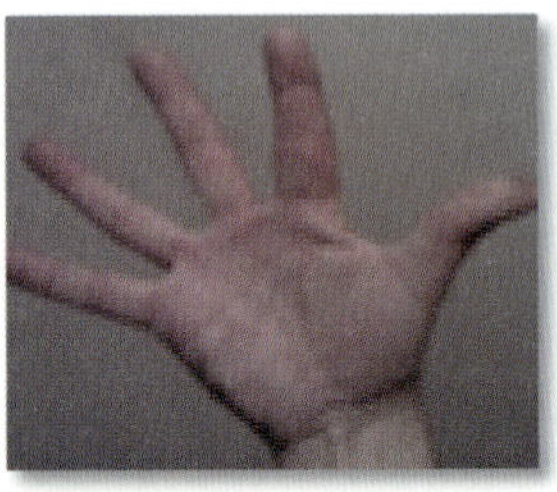

Open your hand: 손을 펴세요

Key Words

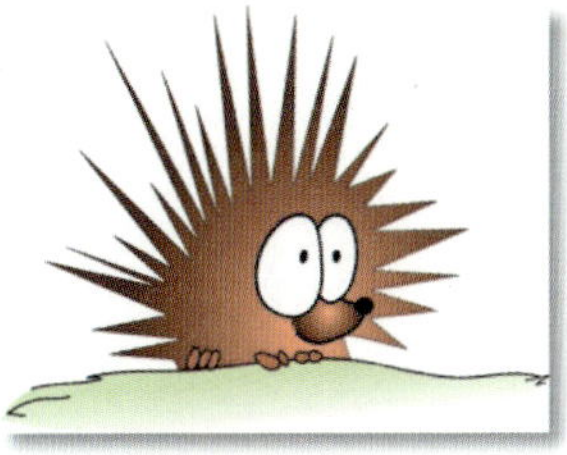

Prick: 따끔함

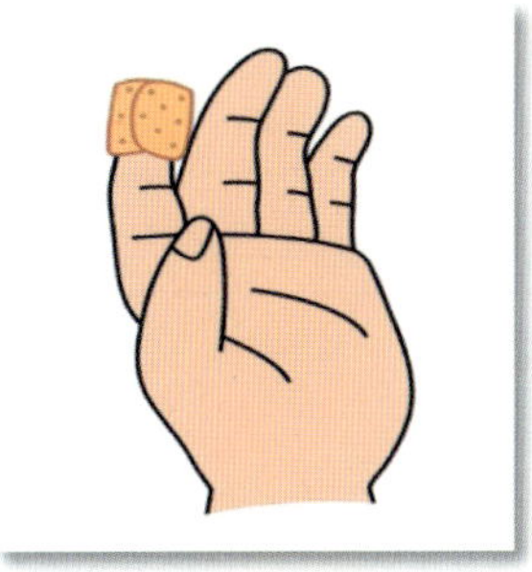

Finger stick blood test
/Finger prick blood test/
Capillary puncture: 손가락 천자 혈액검사

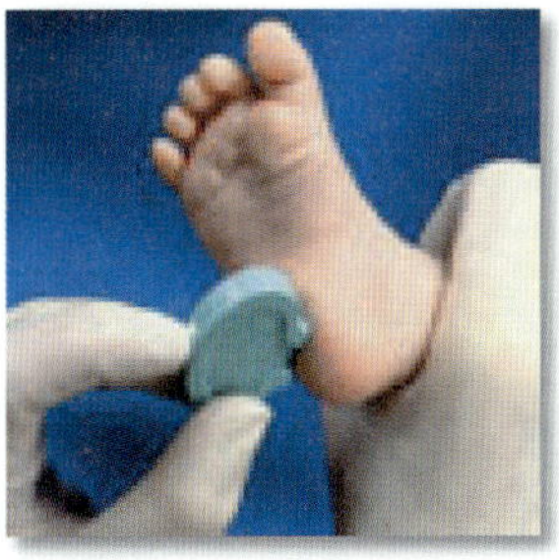

Neonatal heel stick/Neonatal heel prick:
영아 발뒤꿈치 천자 혈액검사

The neonatal heel prick is a common procedure for taking a blood sample from the heel of newborn infants.

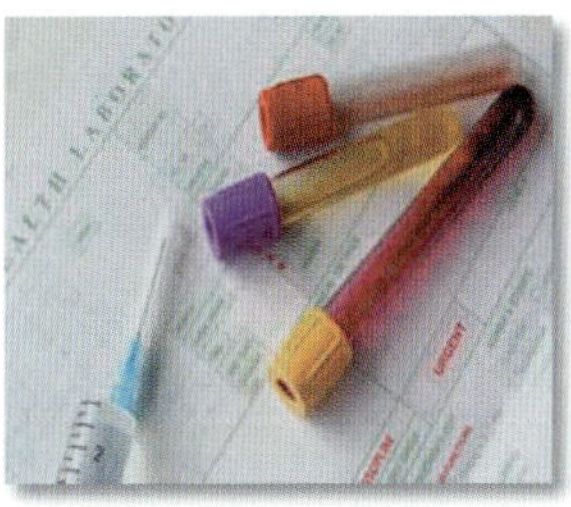

Lab slip: 검사용지
Lab slip for a blood test/Blood test slip:
혈액검사용지

QUIZ: 내 단어장 점검하기 !!

아래 단어를 읽고 알맞은 뜻을 적어보세요.

Finger prick(=stick) blood test: ....

Phlebotomist: ....

Blood drawing room: ....

Blood lab: ....

Blood test vial: ....

Venipuncture blood test: ....

Tourniquet: ....

Make a fist/Make a tight fist: ....

Lab slip: ....

Open your hand: ....

Prick: ....

Capillary puncture: ....

Blood work: ....

Lab slip for a blood test: ....

Blood collection tube: ....

Neonatal heel stick(=prick): ....

Blood test slip: ....

Drill: 아래의 단어를 ***Word Search Puzzle***에서 찾아보세요.

J	S	T	E	D	O	I	R	K	B	W	A	N	B	O
R	V	O	N	V	M	T	N	L	X	A	C	M	L	X
B	V	A	O	V	M	P	O	U	W	F	Y	V	O	E
P	Q	P	S	T	J	O	G	R	C	M	F	F	O	X
K	C	L	K	M	D	C	Y	P	J	P	D	N	D	F
R	J	X	O		V	A	T	Y	F	D	N	U		W
E	U	O	W	T	O	U	R	N	I	Q	U	E	T	O
B	L	O	O	D	L	A	B	B	T	E	T	S	E	G
O	R	D	P	H	L	E	B	O	T	O	M	I	S	T
K	P	J	O	R	L	L	S	F	T	S	O	G	T	E
D	O	T	G	L	I	E	G	A	B	U	W	S		Q
X	E	I	W	U	I	C	P	R	H	R	P	X	S	T
H	O	F	L	X	C	F	K	C	O	A	I	U	L	U
L	U	S	I	X	N	W	G	X	B	N	V	S	I	D
P	L	P	L	O	K	M	V	T	K	C	J	K	P	B

채혈사, 혈액검사실, 토니켓, 따끔함,
혈액검사, 혈액검사용지

Reading material

My Blood Work!

Question:

I have to get a blood test and I have to go and get 3 vials. Is it going to hurt? And is 3 vials a lot?

Answers:

The anticipation of the syringe stick is worse than the actual pain.
Once they've hit your vein, you won't feel any more discomfort.
And it takes less than a second for the phlebotomist or nurse to hit your vein.
BINGO! It's all over.

Ha ha! Trust me. Three vials is nothing. I am the QUEEN of blood tests, and I've had innumerable vials sucked out of me. Three vials is no big deal, and you won't feel any different afterwards.
Don't worry about it! =D
Best of luck!

Words

vial: 혈액을 담는 용기

syringe: 주사

stick: 찌름

vein: 정맥

hit your vein: 정맥에 주사바늘을 놓다

BINGO: 됐다, 바로 그거예요, 맞췄다

QUEEN of something: 무엇인가에 “일가견이 있다” 라는 표현

innumerable: 셀 수 없이 많은

Code Breaker's Corner: 로리와 함께하는 미국 문화 엿보기

What is a Phlebotomist?

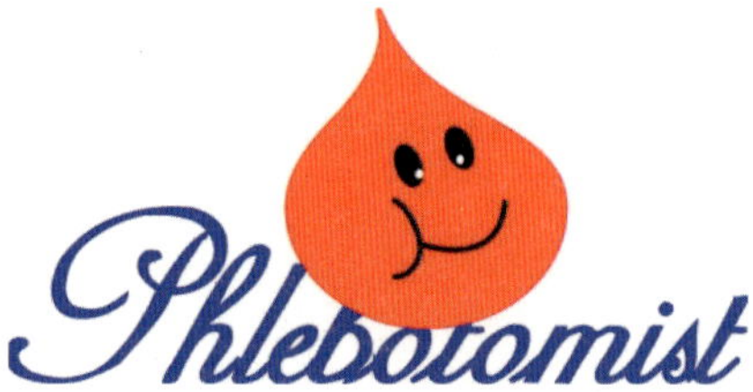

Phlebotomists are medical professionals who draw blood from patients for various lab tests and procedures. A high school graduate or college student could take a course at a local technical or vocational school and learn phlebotomy.

Words

Phlebotomist: 채혈사

medical professional(s): 전문 의료인(들)

take a course: 수업을 듣다.

local technical or vocational school: 지역 내에 있는 직업학교

phlebotomy: 채혈

Facts about Blood Draws

What is a Blood Draw?

A blood draw is a way to collect blood so that lab test can be done to check your health. Each blood draw takes about 5 to 10 minutes. You may resume a normal diet and activities afterwards, although you may experience some soreness for a day or so at the site where the blood was drawn.

Types of Blood Draws

There are two types of blood draws—finger stick/finger prick and venipuncture (VEEN-a-punk-cher). A finger stick/finger prick uses a small needle to prick the fingertip in order to collect a few drops of blood. Venipuncture uses a needle to draw blood out of the vein in your inner arm (forearm).

Home Preparation

No home preparation is needed unless ordered by your doctor. Your doctor may ask you not to eat for a certain amount of time before a blood draw. Please follow the specific instructions given to you by your doctor.

Before the Blood Draw

Blood draws can be done during the doctor's visit (outpatient) or while you are in the hospital. Most outpatient blood draws follow a similar process. After you have checked in at the registration Desk, you will be asked to sit in the waiting area.

During the Blood Draw

You will be joined in the examining room by the nurse or phlebotomist. You will sit in a comfortable chair while the blood draw is being done.

After the Blood Draw

When the nurse or phlebotomist has taken out the needle after all the blood samples needed are collected, the blood draw is over. The nurse or phlebotomist will press on the spot of the venipuncture with alcohol swab and then place the bandage on it. After the procedure, you may resume normal activities. Once the results are in, the doctor will talk about them with you.

Words

blood draw: 채혈

lab test: 기본검사

resume a normal diet: 일반식사를 재개하다

afterwards: 나중에, 그 뒤에

soreness: 통증

finger stick/finger prick: 손가락 천자

venipuncture: 정맥채혈

fingertip: 손가락 끝

inner arm: 팔의 안쪽 부위

doctor's visit (outpatient): 외래진료

check in: 접수하다

waiting area: 대기실

examining room: 검사실

spot: 부위

alcohol swab: 알코올솜

Key Expressions for Blood Work

Wh-Questions~

1. Where should I go for my blood work?
2. When can I get my blood test results back?/ When will the test results come in?
3. What is this test for?

Could I/you~ Would I/you~

4. Could I see your blood test slip please?
5. Could I have your name please?
6. Could you please have a seat and roll up your left sleeve for me?
7. Could you roll up your right sleeve for me?
8. Could you make a tight fist please?

9. **Could you** please put your arm on the table?
10. **Would you** prefer to lie down when I draw the blood from you?
11. **Would you** please not move your arm while I am drawing the blood from your forearm?

Do you ~?
Did you ~?

12. **Do you have** needle phobia?
13. **Do you have** trypanophobia?
14. **Do you have** any questions for your blood test?
15. **Did you** eat anything before the test?

Others

16. **Is it going to hurt?**

17. Are there any dietary restrictions for me to prepare for my blood test?
18. Have you ever passed out when you had a blood test before?
19. How long does it normally take to get blood work results back?
20. You can open your fist now.
21. It is all over./We are all finished now.
22. This rubber cord/tourniquet/elastic band may feel tight.
23. I am going to tie a rubber cord around the upper part of your arm to make the veins Bulge slightly.
24. I am going to place a tourniquet on your upper arm to make your veins more noticeable.
25. I am going to insert the needle in a slanted position and blood will be drawn into a vial.

Words

left sleeve: 왼쪽 소매

make a tight fist: 주먹을 꽉 쥐세요

lie down: 눕다

forearm: 전완

trypanophobia: 주사공포증

dietary restrictions: 식사제한

pass out: 실신하다

fist: 주먹

open your fist: 주먹을 펴세요

rubber cord: 압박 고무줄

bulge: 튀어나온, 불거지게

noticeable: 눈에 두드러진

slanted: 비스듬히

Drill: Q1-Q25를 영작하세요.

정답은 전 페이지의 Key Expressions for Blood Work를 참고하세요.

Q1. 혈액검사를 받으러 어디로 가야 하나요? ____________________

____

Q2. 언제 혈액검사 결과를 알 수 있을까요?/검사 결과를 언제 알 수 있을까요? ____________________

____

Q3. 이것은 무슨 검사인가요?

____

Q4. 혈액검사용지를 볼 수 있을까요?

____

Q5. 성함이 무엇입니까?

____

Q6. 자리에 앉으시고 왼쪽 소매를 올려주시겠습니까?

____

Q7. 오른쪽 소매를 올려주시겠습니까?

____

Q8. 주먹을 꽉 쥐시겠습니까? ....

Q9. 팔을 이 테이블 위에 올려주시겠습니까?

....

Q10. 채혈을 할 때 누우시는 것이 더 나을까요?

....

Q11. 팔에서 채혈을 하는 동안 움직이지 마세요.

....

Q12. 바늘에 대한 공포증이 있습니까?

....

Q13. 주사공포증이 있습니까?

....

Q14. 혈액검사에 관한 질문사항이 있습니까?

....

Q15. 검사 전에 먹은 것이 있나요?

....

Q16. 아플까요?

....

Q17. 검사 전에 제한해야 할 음식이 있습니까?

....

Q18. 혈액검사를 받을 때 실신한 적이 있습니까?

Q19. 혈액검사 결과를 받으려면 보통 얼마나 걸리나요?

Q20. 이제 주먹을 펴도 됩니다.

Q21. 다 끝났습니다./이제 다 끝났습니다.

Q22. 이 압박고무줄/토니켓/고무밴드가 조일 것입니다.

Q23. 핏줄을 더 잘 드러나게 하기 위해 팔의 윗 부분을 압박고무줄로 감겠습니다.

Q24. 핏줄이 더 잘 드러나게 하기 위해 팔뚝에 토니켓을 감겠습니다.

Q25. 바늘은 비스듬하게 들어가고 혈액은 용기에 담길 것입니다.

2. Cholesterol Test/Lipid Panel Test
콜레스테롤검사/지질검사

- **Needle Phobia, 바늘 공포증**
  - Words, 어휘
- **Cholesterol Test/Lipid Panel Test, 콜레스테롤검사/지질검사**
  - Words, 어휘
- **Story of My Blood Work, 나의 혈액검사 이야기**
  - Dialogue: Cholesterol Test, 대화: 콜레스테롤 검사
  - Words, 어휘
  - Review, 복습문제

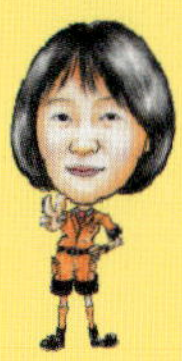

이 책의 녹음 파일은 www.ohgieun.com 에서 무료다운로드 하실 수 있습니다

Needle Phobia!

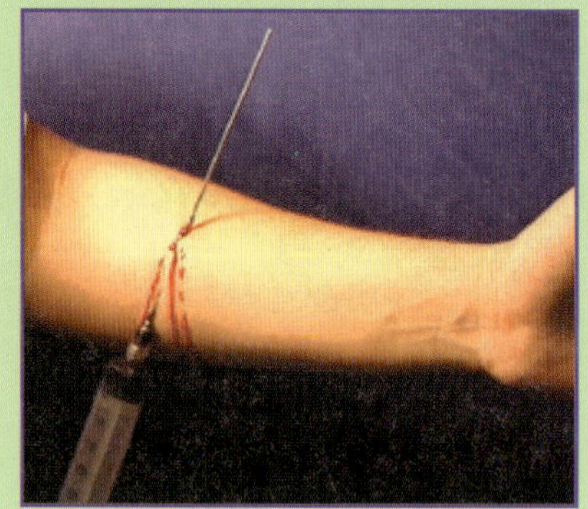

www.magic.org

Today, the diagnostic process as well as preventive medicine regularly includes both injections and blood testing, both that require needles. However, approximately 10% of the population has needle phobia, or an intense fear of needles and sharp objects. People with needle phobia often report an immense amount of pain associated with receiving an injection or having to have blood tested. Needle phobia can be dangerous, not only because of the direct physical symptoms that occur, but because people will avoid medical care because of their fear.

Needle phobia was once thought to be an emotional response to needles and a childhood fear. However, according to an article, “Needle Phobia: The Neglected Diagnosis”, by Dr. James G. Hamilton, this condition is “not confined to children, is not an emotion-driven or transient phenomenon, and is not a rare condition.” Dr. Hamilton explains that physicians must be aware and conscious of the condition, because “it is a common condition and because needle-phobic persons tend to avoid medical treatment, which can lead to serious health problems as well as social and legal problems.”

There are several different phobias which fear of needles can fall under:

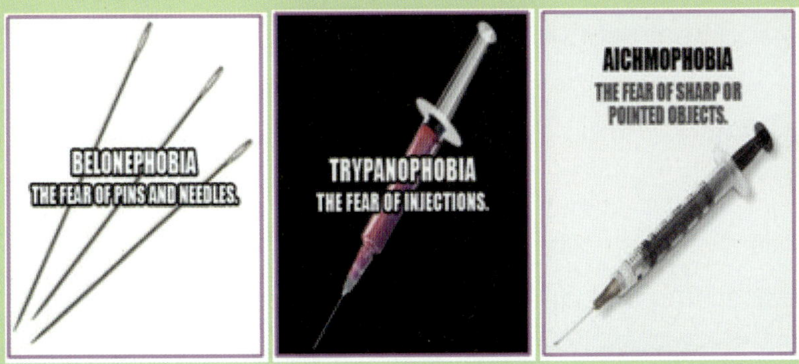

weirdphobia.com

Belonephobia: The fear of pins and needles.

Trypanophobia: The fear of injections.

Aichmophobia: The fear of sharp or pointed objects.

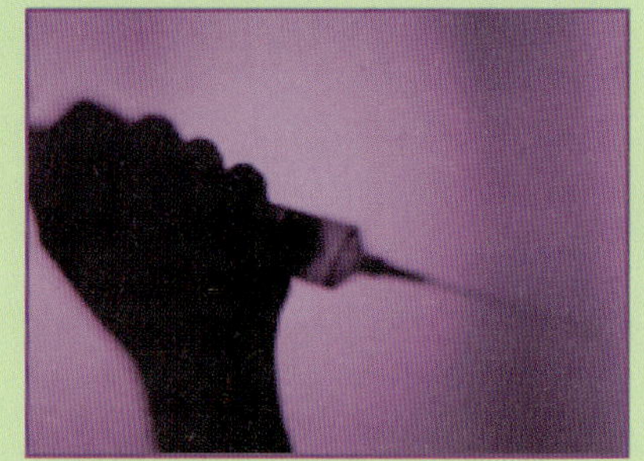

Symptoms

Physical symptoms, such as the rise in blood pressure (hypertension), increase in heart rate (tachycardia), and increase in stress hormones, dizziness and possible loss of consciousness (vasovagal reflex) are measurable even at the thought of having an injection or blood testing. Therefore, it should be considered and addressed to help a patient when needles are a necessary part of medical treatment.

Treatment

While many anxiety disorders are treated with a combination of medication and cognitive behavioral therapy, this treatment does not seem to improve needle phobia. For people with this type of phobia, talking with your doctor about some of the methods below may help to alleviate the symptoms:

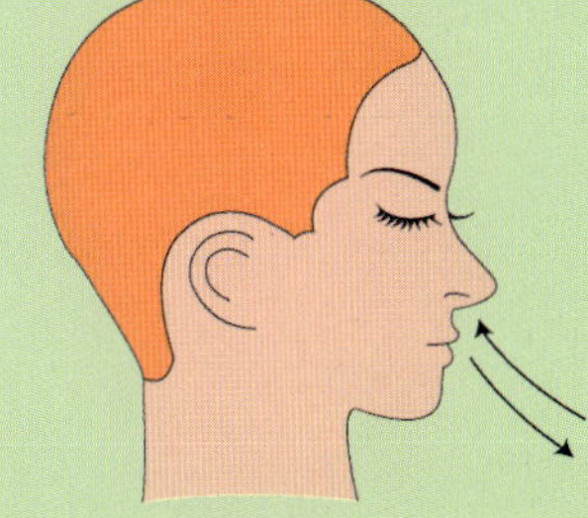

Body positioning

Dizziness and loss of consciousness can be a serious concern. These symptoms are lessened when a patient lies with their feet elevated and their head down while receiving an injection or needle. Patients should remain in this position until they feel comfortable and should very slowly move to a sitting or standing position.

Behavioral Strategies

Talk with the doctor or medical professional before receiving an injection and discuss your needle phobia. Make sure the medical professional is experienced and skilled at giving injections or taking blood. Breathe slowly and deeply while having an injection or having blood drawn. This can help to reduce other physical symptoms.

References:
"Needle Phobia", 2007, Jerry Emanualson, NeedlePhobia.com
"Needle Phobia: The Neglected Diagnosis", 1995, James G. Hamilton, M.D., Journal of Family Practice
"Needle Phobia Information", Date Unknown, D. Keith Lamb, The Needle Phobia Information Site http://www.healthcentral.com/anxiety/disorder-types-273889-5.html

Words

preventive medicine: 예방의학

injection: 주사

immense: 상당한

emotion-driven: 감정에 의한

transient phenomenon: 일시적인 현상

belonephobia: 핀과 바늘에 대한 공포증

trypanophobia: 주사공포증

aichmophobia: 예리하고 날카로운 물건에 대한 공포증

hypertension: 고혈압

tachycardia: 빈맥

dizziness: 어지럼증

loss of consciousness: 의식을 잃음

vasovagal reflex: 혈관미주신경반사

anxiety disorders: 불안장애

cognitive behavioral therapy: 인지활동치료

alleviate: 완화시키다

behavioral strategies: 행동전략

medical professional: 전문의료인

experienced and skilled: 경험이 있고 숙련된

breathe slowly and deeply: 천천히 길게 숨을 쉬다

Cholesterol Test/ Lipid Panel Test

The Cholesterol Test/Lipid Panel Test, also called a coronary risk profile, is a group of tests used to help determine risk of coronary heart disease.

Cholesterol Test (=Lipid Panel Test) measures **Total cholesterol**, **Triglycerides, HDL,** and **LDL.**

Total cholesterol is the sum of the different types of cholesterols.

Triglycerides store energy until the body needs it. When you eat too many calories your body makes triglycerides, the storage form of fat. If the body holds on to too much triglycerides, blood vessels can get clogged and cause health problems.

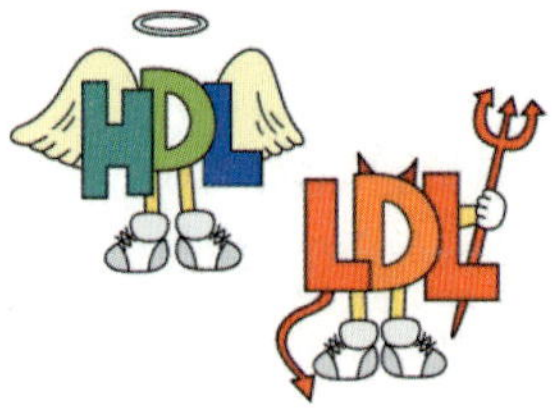

High-Density Lipoproteins (HDL) cholesterol is commonly called "good" cholesterol. High-density lipoproteins carry cholesterol from the blood streams to the liver to be eliminated.

Low-Density Lipoproteins (LDL) cholesterol is commonly known as "bad" cholesterol. Low-density lipoproteins that build up in the bloodstream can clog blood vessels and increase the risk of heart disease.

Words

Lipid Panel Test: 지질검사

coronary risk profile: 관상동맥질환 고 위험군

Total cholesterol: 총콜레스테롤

Triglycerides: 중성지방

High-Density Lipoproteins (HDL) cholesterol: 고밀도 지단백질 콜레스테롤

Low-Density Lipoproteins (LDL) cholesterol: 저밀도 지단백질 콜레스테롤

Story of My Blood Work

Cholesterol Test

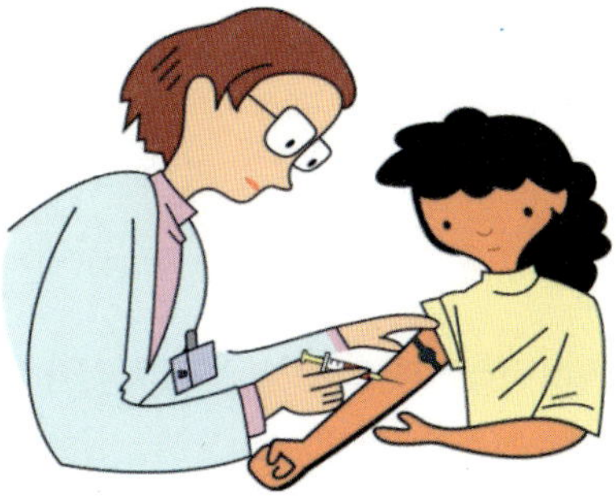

Nurse: Ms. Anderson.

Here is your blood test slip. A phlebotomist will tell you what to do and draw some blood.

Ms. Anderson: Okay. Where should I go for my blood work?

Nurse: Your medical coordinator will take you there.

Ms. Anderson: That's perfect.

Medical coordinator: Hello, Ms. Anderson. I am your medical coordinator, Emily. I will show you the way to the blood lab. Please come this way.

Ms. Anderson: Thank you.

Medical coordinator: No problem.

At The Registration Desk

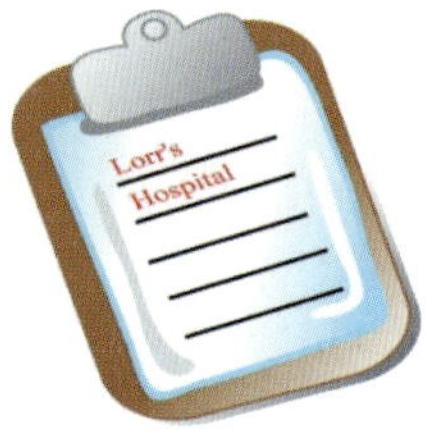

Medical coordinator: Hello. Her doctor sent her over here to have her blood drawn.

Lab Assistant: I can help her with that. Could I see her blood test slip please?

Ms. Anderson: Sure. Here you are.

Lab Assistant: Well, today your doctor wants us to do the Cholesterol Test. Your phlebotomist will be here in a moment.

Ms. Anderson: I see.

Phlebotomist: Hello. I am your phlebotomist. I am going to draw some blood from your forearm. I need to verify a couple of things first. Could I have your name and date of birth please?

Ms. Anderson: Sunny Anderson and February 25th, 1972.

Phlebotomist: Alright, Ms. Anderson. Do you think you have a needle phobia? What I mean is that when you have a blood test or receive an injection, do you feel unreasonably fearful for a needle?

Ms. Anderson: Not that I know of.

Phlebotomist: Good then. Would you please have a seat and roll up your left sleeve for me?

Ms. Anderson: Like this?

Phlebotomist: That's right.

Ms. Anderson: I'm kind of nervous.

Phlebotomist: It will only feel like a little pin prick. So, don't worry about it too much. I will briefly explain the procedure for your blood test. First of all, I am going to put a tourniquet on your upper arm to puff your veins up, and you will feel a little tight around your upper arm.

Ms. Anderson: I see.

Phlebotomist: Then, I am going to wash the area inside your elbow with an antiseptic swab to draw the blood from your forearm. After I put a needle into the vein in your forearm, I will attach test tubes to the needle to collect the blood.

Ms. Anderson: Okay. By the way, how many vials of blood do you need from me?

Phlebotomist: I am going to draw one vial of blood from your forearm. One more thing, when I draw the blood, if you look the other way and remain very still, it will be very helpful. Are you ready now?

Ms. Anderson: Yes, I am.

Phlebotomist: You may feel discomfort by the needle.

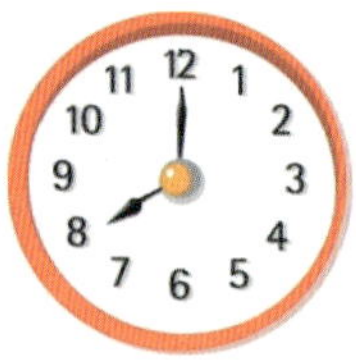

1 minute later

Phlebotomist: There we go! I got the blood that I needed. Now, I will put gauze on the puncture mark, and you need to apply pressure on it to stop the blood flow, but you shouldn't rub it. Please bend your arm to assist the process. Do you have any questions before you leave?

Ms. Anderson: Um. Am I going to have bruise at the puncture mark?

Phlebotomist: You might expect possible bruising to occur at the wound site as well as a bit of pain.

Ms. Anderson: I see. I have another question for you. When can I get my blood test results back?

Phlebotomist: It takes about a week. When the result is sent to your doctor, we will let you know as soon as possible.

Ms. Anderson: Thank you!

Phlebotomist: No problem. Thank you for coming in today.

Words

blood test slip: 혈액검사용지

draw some blood: 채혈을 하다

blood work=blood test: 혈액검사

needle phobia: 바늘 공포증

pin prick: 핀으로 찌르는 듯한

antiseptic swab: 소독약이 묻은 솜

forearm: 전완

vial: 혈액 검사 용기

remain very still: 전혀 움직이지 않고 있다

puncture mark: 채혈을 한 부위

blood flow: 피가 흐르는

bruise: 멍

*** 1 vial is 5 to 7cc.**
cc=cubic centimeter

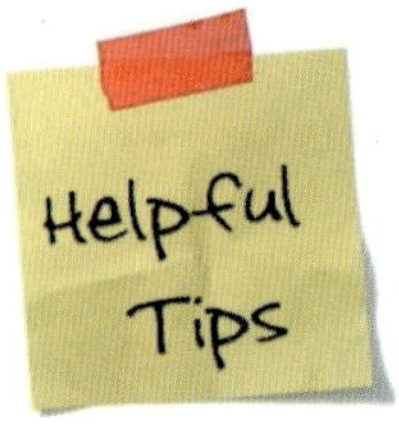

Understanding Cholesterol Numbers:
콜레스테롤검사 수치

Total Cholesterol	**Under 200**	Desirable
	200 - 239	Borderline High
	Over 240	High
HDL Cholesterol The GOOD kind	**Over 60**	Optimal
	Under 40	Low for Men
	Under 50	Low for Women
LDL Cholesterol The BAD kind - a lower number is better	**Under 70**	Optimal for those with heart or blood vessel disease
	Under 100	Optimal (also for diabetics & those with risk factors for heart disease)
	100 - 129	Near Optimal
	130 - 159	Borderline High
	160 - 189	High
	Over 190	Very High
Triglycerides	**Under 150**	Normal
	150 - 199	Borderline High
	200 - 499	High
	Over 500	Very High

Resource: www.cholesterollevelschart.net

Review 각각의 구문을 영작하세요.
정답은 전 페이지의 Dialogue를 참고하세요.

Nurse: Ms. Anderson.

여기 혈액검사용지가 있습니다. ....

채혈사가 무엇을 해야 하는지 알려줄 것이고 채혈을 할 것입니다.

....

Ms. Anderson: 알겠습니다. 혈액검사 받으러 어디로 가야 하나요? ....

Nurse: Your medical coordinator will take you there.

Ms. Anderson: That's perfect.

Medical coordinator: Hello, Ms. Anderson. I am your medical coordinator, Emily.

제가 혈액검사실로 안내해 드리겠습니다. 이쪽으로 오세요. ....

....

Ms. Anderson: Thank you.

Medical coordinator: No problem.

At The Registration Desk

Medical coordinator: 안녕하세요. 이 환자분의 의사선생님이 혈액검사를 하라고 이곳으로 보냈습니다. ....

....

Lab Assistant: 제가 도와드리겠습니다. 환자분의 혈액검사용지를 볼 수 있을까요? ....

....

Ms. Anderson: Sure. Here you are.

Lab Assistant: 환자분의 주치의가 콜레스테롤 검사를 처방하셨습니다. ....

채혈사가 곧 올 것입니다. ....

Ms. Anderson: I see.

Phlebotomist: Hello. I am your phlebotomist.

제가 환자의 팔(전완)에서 채혈을 하겠습니다. ....

....

우선 몇 가지 확인을 하겠습니다. ....

환자분의 성함과 생년월일을 말씀해 주시겠습니까? ....

....

Ms. Anderson: Sunny Anderson and February 25th, 1972.

Phlebotomist: Alright, Ms. Anderson.

바늘에 대한 공포증이 있습니까? 제 말은 혈액검사를 받거나 주사를 맞을 때, 주사바늘에 대한 이해할 수 없을 정도의 공포를 느끼나요? ....

....

Ms. Anderson: Not that I know of.

Phlebotomist: Good then.

앉으셔서 왼쪽 소매를 걷어주시겠습니까? ....

....

Ms. Anderson: Like this?

Phlebotomist: That's right.

Ms. Anderson: I'm kind of nervous.

Phlebotomist: It will only feel like a little pin prick. So, don't worry about it too much.

제가 간단하게 진행절차를 설명해 드리겠습니다. ....

....

우선 팔의 정맥이 좀더 잘 나타나게 하기 위해 팔의 윗 부분에 토니켓을 감겠습니다. ....

....

조금 조이는 듯한 느낌을 받을 것입니다. ....

....

Ms. Anderson: I see.

Phlebotomist: 그런 후, 채혈하기 위해 팔꿈치의 안쪽 부위를 소독솜으로 닦겠습니다. ....

....

제가 주사바늘을 꽂은 후에 혈액을 담기 위해 튜브를 바늘에 연결할 것입니다. ....

....

Ms. Anderson: Okay. By the way, how many vials of blood do you need from me?

Phlebotomist: 튜브 1개를 채혈할 것입니다. ....

....

한 가지 더요. 제가 채혈을 할 때 다른 곳을 보고 움직이지 않으면 도움이 되실 것입니다. ....

....

Are you ready now?

Ms. Anderson: Yes, I am.

Phlebotomist: You may feel discomfort by the needle.

1 minute later

Phlebotomist: There we go! I got the blood that I needed.

이제 채혈한 부위에 거즈를 대겠습니다. 지혈이 되도록 누르시면 됩니다. 하지만 문지르면 안됩니다.

지혈을 돕기 위해 팔을 굽혀주세요.

Do you have any questions before you leave?

Ms. Anderson: Um. Am I going to have bruise at the puncture mark?

Phlebotomist: 아마도 멍이 들 수도 있고 조금 아플 수도 있습니다.

Ms. Anderson: I see. I have another question for you.
When can I get my blood test results back?

Phlebotomist: It takes about a week.

결과가 환자분의 담당의사에게 전해지면 즉시 알려드리겠습니다.

Ms. Anderson: Thank you!

Phlebotomist: No problem. Thank you for coming in today.

3. Complete Blood Count (CBC)Test
전혈구 검사

- **Complete Blood Count (CBC) Test, 전혈구 검사**
  - Words, 어휘

- **Story of My Blood Work, 나의 혈액검사 이야기**
  - Dialogue: STAT Order! Complete Blood Count Test, 대화: 긴급검사! 전혈구 검사
  - Words, 어휘
  - Review, 복습문제

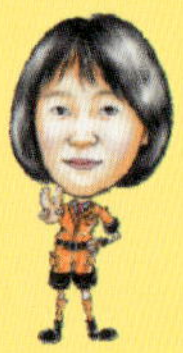

이 책의 녹음 파일은 www.ohgieun.com 에서 무료다운로드 하실 수 있습니다

Complete Blood Count(CBC) Test

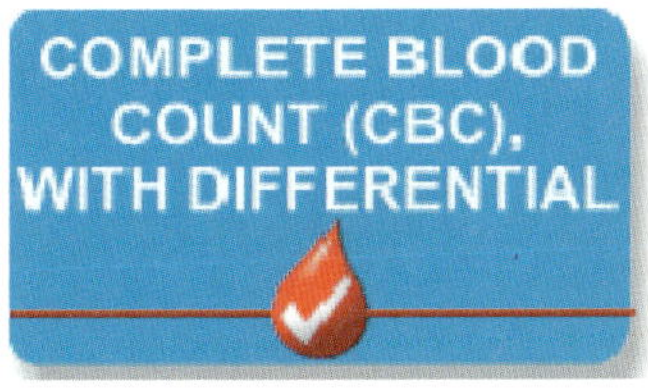

The CBC is a very common test. Many patients will have baseline CBC tests to help determine their general health status. The CBC is used as a broad screening test to check for disorders such as anemia, infection, and many other diseases. It is actually a panel of tests that examines different parts of the blood such as the number of red blood cells (RBCs), the number of white blood cells (WBCs), the total amount of hemoglobin in the blood and others.

Words

CBC: 전혈구 검사
broad screening test: 판별검사
anemia: 빈혈
infection: 감염
a panel of tests: 전반적인 검사
red blood cell: 적혈구
white blood cell: 백혈구

Story of My Blood Work

STAT Order! Complete Blood Count Test

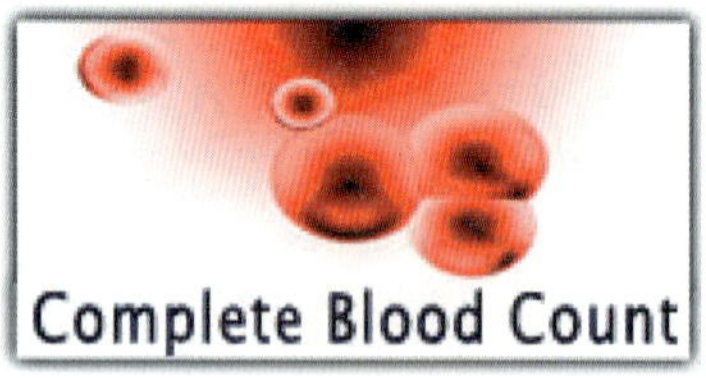

Lab Assistant: Could I have your name please?

Patient: Ken Johnson.

Lab Assistant: Okay, Mr. Johnson. Could I see your blood work order slip please?

Mr. Johnson: Here it is. What is this test for?

Lab Assistant: Well, today your doctor ordered CBC test to check your white blood cell count.

Mr. Johnson: What does my white blood cell count tell my doctor?

Lab Assistant: If it is elevated, you might have an infection.

Mr. Johnson: Oh, I see.

Lab Assistant: Have a seat and sign your name at the bottom of this paper please.

Mr. Johnson: Alright.

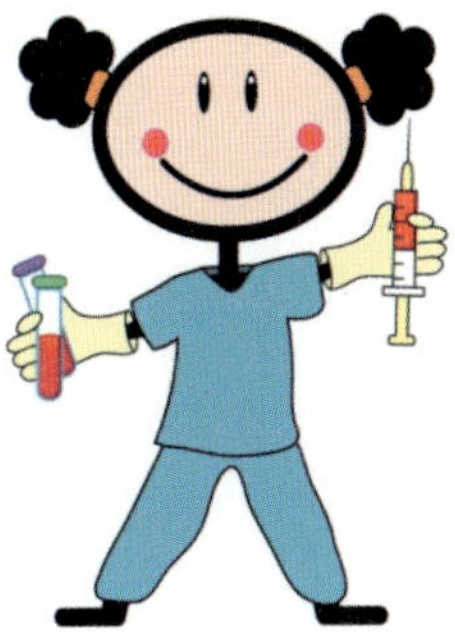

Lab Assistant: Emily, we have a patient. His doctor put a STAT order on it. We need his blood work STAT. Can you draw the blood from him right now?

Emily (Phlebotomist): Sure. I'll do it right away.

Lab Assistant: I really appreciate your prompt response.

Emily (Phlebotomist): Oh, no problem.

Emily(Phlebotomist): Hello. I am your phlebotomist. First of all, could I have your name and DOB please?

Mr. Johnson: Ken Johnson and May 30th, 1970.

Emily (Phlebotomist): Thank you, Mr. Johnson. I am going to draw some blood from your arm. Please roll up your right sleeve for me.

Mr. Johnson: Um. I am right-handed, so I have always had my blood drawn from my left arm. Can you do it on my left arm instead?

Emily (Phlebotomist): Sure. No problem at all. Anything else?

Mr. Johnson: Nope.

Emily (Phlebotomist): Then, please roll up your left sleeve for me.

Mr. Johnson: Okay.

Emily (Phlebotomist): Please straighten your arm. I will wrap this tourniquet around your upper arm and disinfect your arm with alcohol swab.

Mr. Johnson: I see.

Emily (Phlebotomist): Please make a tight fist for three times and hold your squeeze on the last one.

Mr. Johnson: Okay.

Emily (Phlebotomist): You will feel just a little prick, but it does not hurt much. Please hold still while I am taking the blood.

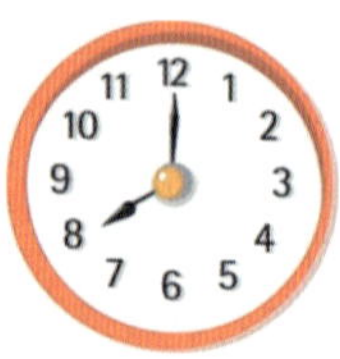

2 minutes later

Emily (Phlebotomist): Well, we are all finished. You can open your hand. Press on this cotton pad against the area, but don't rub it please. Bend your arm for five minutes, please.
Mr. Johnson: Okay.

Emily (Phlebotomist): It will take around 40 minutes to get your blood work results back. When the results have come in, your doctor will discuss the test results with you. For now, you can wait in the waiting area.
Mr. Johnson: Alright. Thank you.

Words

STAT: 긴급한 검사

blood work order slip=blood work test slip: 혈액검사용지

appreciate: 감사합니다

prompt response: 빠른 응대

roll up: ~을 걷어 올리다

right-handed: 오른손잡이

alcohol swab: 알코올 소독 솜

make a tight fist: 주먹을 꽉 쥐세요

prick: 조금 따끔하다

open your hand: 손을 펴다

cotton pad: 솜

against the area: 그 부위에 대고

waiting area: 대기실

Review 각각의 구문을 영작하세요.
정답은 전 페이지의 Dialogue를 참고하세요.

Lab Assistant: Could I have your name please?

Patient: Ken Johnson.

Lab Assistant: Okay, Mr. Johnson.

혈액검사용지를 보여주시겠습니까? ....

....

Mr. Johnson: 여기 있습니다. 무슨 검사인가요? ....

....

Lab Assistant: Well, today your doctor ordered CBC test to check your white blood cell count.

Mr. Johnson: What does my white blood cell count tell my doctor?

Lab Assistant: 만일 백혈구 수치가 올라가면 염증이 있다는

것을 말합니다. ....

....

Mr. Johnson: Oh, I see.

Lab Assistant: 여기에 앉으시고 이 서류의 하단에 서명해 주세요. ....

....

Mr. Johnson: Alright.

Lab Assistant: Emily, we have a patient.
환자의 담당의사가 긴급검사로 지시를 내렸습니다. ....

....

이 환자의 혈액검사를 급히 해야 합니다. 지금 이 환자의 채혈을 해 주시겠습니까? ....

....

Emily (Phlebotomist): Sure. I'll do it right away.

Lab Assistant: I really appreciate your prompt response.
Emily (Phlebotomist): Oh, no problem.

Emily (Phlebotomist): Hello. I am your phlebotomist. First of all, could I have your name and DOB please?
Mr. Johnson: Ken Johnson and May 30th, 1970.

Emily (Phlebotomist): Thank you, Mr. Johnson.
팔에서 채혈을 하겠습니다. 오른쪽 소매를 걷어주세요. ....

....

Mr. Johnson: Um. I am right-handed, so I have always had my blood drawn from my left arm. Can you do it on my left arm instead?

Emily (Phlebotomist): Sure. No problem at all. Anything else?
Mr. Johnson: Nope.

Emily (Phlebotomist): Then, please roll up your left sleeve for me.
Mr. Johnson: Okay.

Emily (Phlebotomist): 팔을 쭉 펴주세요. ....

상완을 토니켓으로 묶고 알코올 솜으로 팔을 소독하겠습니다.

....

Mr. Johnson: I see.

Emily (Phlebotomist): 주먹을 세 번 꽉 쥐세요 그리고 마지막 번에서 주먹을 꽉 쥔 채로 계세요. ....

....

Mr. Johnson: Okay.

Emily(Phlebotomist): 조금 따끔해요. 그러나 많이 아프지는 않아요. ....

제가 채혈하는 동안에 움직이지 마세요. ....

....

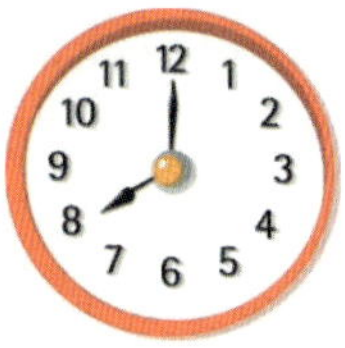

2 minutes later

Emily (Phlebotomist): 다 끝났습니다. 주먹을 펴도 됩니다.

채혈한 부위에 솜을 대고 누르세요.

하지만 문지르시면 안 되요.

약 5 분 동안 팔을 굽히고 계세요.

Mr. Johnson: Okay.

Emily (Phlebotomist): 혈액검사 결과는 약 40분 가량 걸립니다.

결과가 나오면 의사선생님과 함께 상의 하실 것입니다.

그 동안 대기실에서 기다려 주세요.

Mr. Johnson: Alright. Thank you.

4. Finger Prick/Finger Stick Blood Test
손가락 천자 혈액검사

- **Finger Prick/Finger Stick Blood Test, 손가락 천자 혈액검사**
  - Words, 어휘
- **Story of My Blood Work, 나의 혈액검사 이야기**
  - Dialogue: Jenny's Finger Prick Blood Test, 제니의 손가락 천자 혈액검사
  - Words, 어휘
  - Review, 복습문제

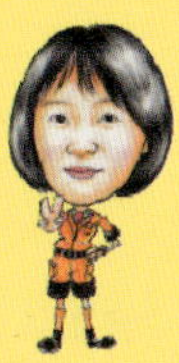

이 책의 녹음 파일은 www.ohgieun.com 에서 무료다운로드 하실 수 있습니다

Finger Prick/Finger Stick Blood Test

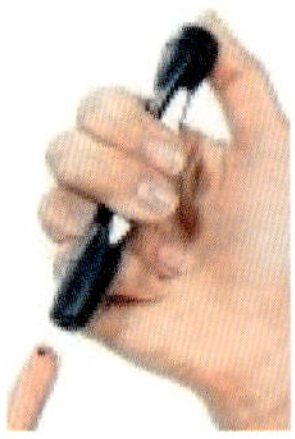

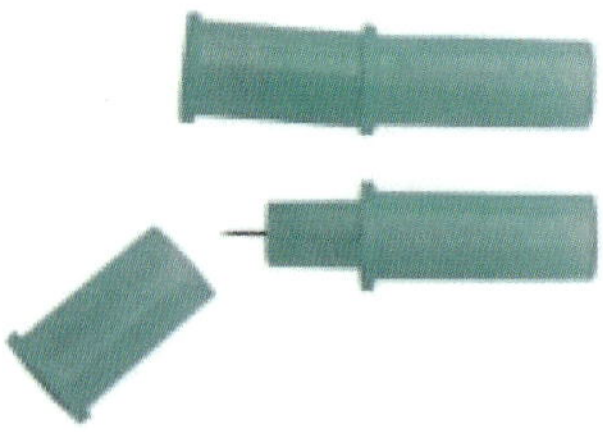

Lancet

In infants or young children, a sharp tool called a lancet may be used to puncture the skin and make it bleed. The blood collects into a capillary tube.

Words

finger prick/finger stick blood test: 손가락 천자 혈액검사

infant: 영아

sharp tool: 예리한 도구

puncture: 구멍을 내다

capillary tube: 모세관

Story of My Blood Work

Jenny's Finger Prick Blood Test

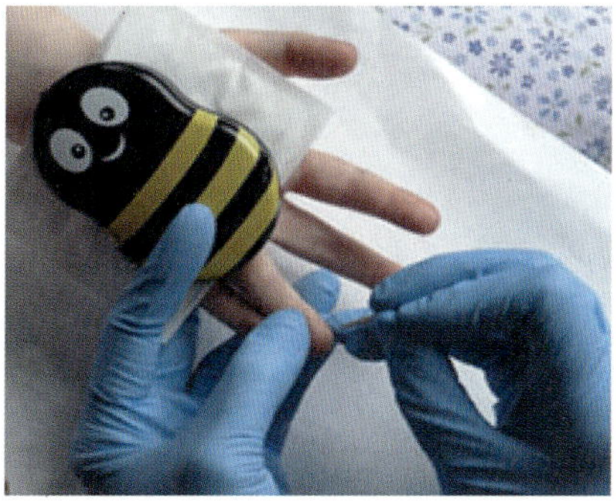

Patient's parent: My daughter has an appointment for blood test today.

Nurse: I see. What's her name and date of birth please?

Patient's parent: Jenny Smith and 07/09/2002.

Nurse: Alright. Hello, Jenny! Have a seat please.

Jenny: Okay.

Nurse: I am going to draw very small amount of blood from your finger today. First, I am going to swab your fingertip with alcohol.

Jenny: Which finger do you need?

Nurse: I would like to have your middle or ring finger please.

Jenny: How about my pinky?

Nurse: Your pinky is not suitable for the test because the fifth finger does not have sufficient tissue to prevent the bone injury.

Jenny: Oh, I didn't know that. Then I will have it done on my middle finger.

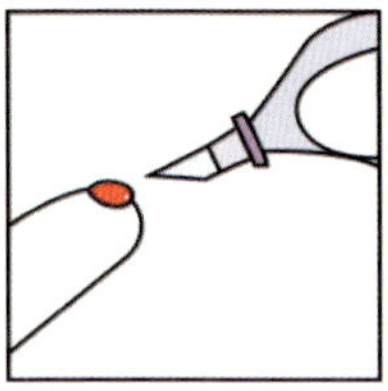

Nurse: Good. This is called lancet. I am going to use this lancet to produce blood from your fingertip.

Jenny: Does it hurt?

Nurse: Just a little prick. Like a bee sting. Do you need your mom to hold you?

Jenny: Yes. Please.

Nurse: Ma'am. You can hold your daughter.

Jenny's mom: Alright.

Nurse: Jenny. I will hold your middle finger downward position and poke the fingertip. Ready?

Jenny: Yes.

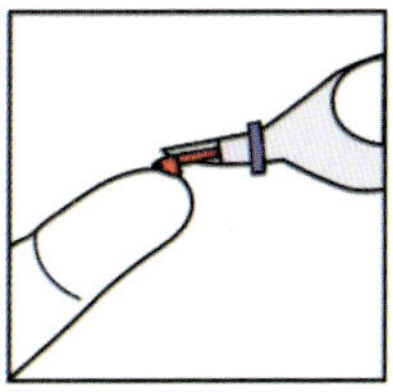

Nurse: There we go. Poking part is over. I will put the capillary tube on the fingertip to collect the blood.

Jenny: It didn't hurt much.

Nurse: I told you. Well, the tube is filled now. The test is over and I'll place a very cute band-aid on your finger. You can remove your band-aid later today or the next morning.

Jenny: Okay.

Nurse: Thank you for coming in today. See you later alligator.

Words

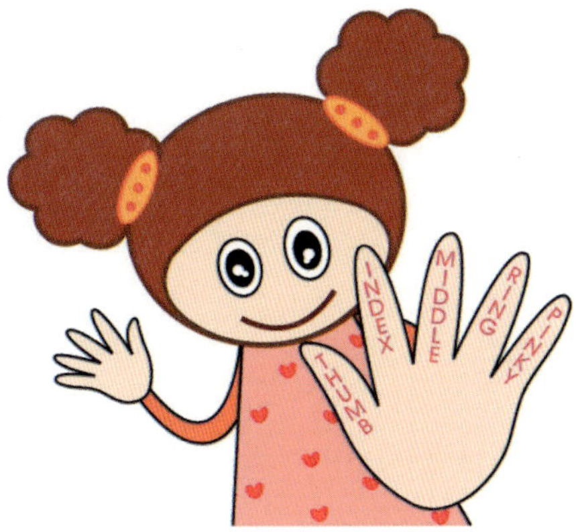

fingertip: 손가락 끝

middle finger: 중지

ring finger: 약지

pinky/baby finger: 새끼 손가락

sufficient tissue: 충분한 조직

bee sting: 벌침

downward: 아래로 향하게

capillary tube: 모세관

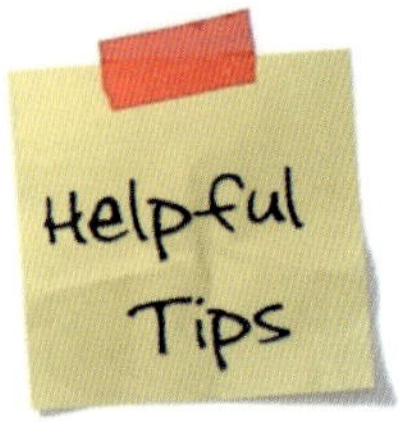

Finger Names: 손가락 명칭

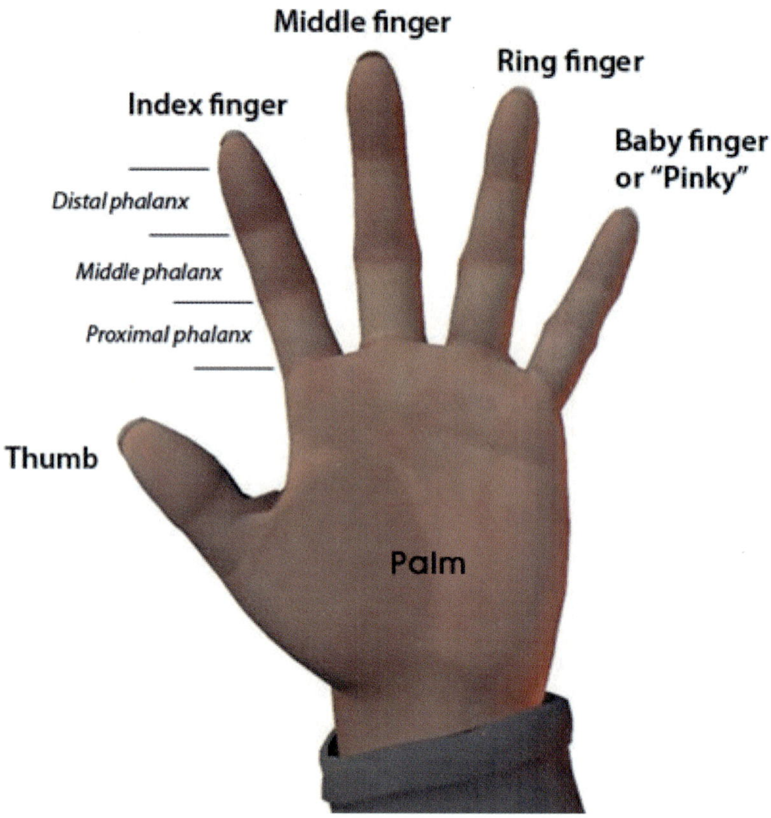

Distal phalanx: 끝 마디 손가락 뼈

Middle phalanx: 중간 마디 손가락 뼈

Proximal phalanx: 첫 마디 손가락뼈

Review 각각의 구문을 영작하세요.
정답은 전 페이지의 Dialogue를 참고하세요.

Patient's parent: 오늘이 딸아이의 혈액검사 예약을 한날입니다.

....

Nurse: 알겠습니다. 이름과 생년월일은 무엇입니까? ....

....

Patient's parent: Jenny Smith and 07/09/2002.

Nurse: Alright. Hello, Jenny! Have a seat please.

Jenny: Okay.

Nurse: 손가락에서 아주 작은 양의 혈액을 채취할 거예요. ....

....

먼저, 손가락 끝을 알코올로 소독하겠습니다. ....

....

Jenny: Which finger do you need?

Nurse: 세 번째 또는 네 번째 손가락에서 혈액검사를 하고 싶은 데요. ....

Jenny: How about my pinky?

Nurse: 새끼 손가락은 검사에 적합하지 않아요. 왜냐하면 손가락 뼈가 다치는 것을 방지할 조직이 충분하지 않아서요.

Jenny: Oh, I didn't know that. Then I will have it done on my middle finger.

Nurse: Good. This is called lancet.

란싯을 사용해서 손가락 끝에서 혈액을 채취할게요.

Jenny: Does it hurt?

Nurse: 조금 따끔해요. 벌침처럼.

엄마보고 안아 달라고 할까요?

Jenny: Yes. Please.

Nurse: 들어오셔서 아이를 안아주세요.

Jenny's mom: Alright.

Nurse: 제니. 세번째 손가락을 아래로 향하게 잡고 손가락 끝에 콕 할게요. 준비됐나요?

Jenny: Yes.

Nurse: 다 됐어요. 찌르는 부분은 끝났어요.

혈액을 수집하기 위해 모세관을 손가락 끝에 댈게요.

Jenny: It didn't hurt much.

Nurse: I told you.

튜브가 다 채워졌어요.

검사가 다 끝났습니다. 그리고 아주 귀여운 반창고를 손가락에 붙여줄게요.

반창고는 오늘 이따가 떼거나 아니면 내일 떼어요.

Jenny: Okay.

Nurse: Thank you for coming in today. See you later alligator.

5. Oral Glucose Tolerance Test
경구당부하검사

- **Oral Glucose Tolerance Test, 경구당부하검사**
  - Words, 어휘
- **Story of My Blood Work, 나의 혈액검사 이야기**
  - Dialogue: Gestational Diabetes Screening Test, 임신성 당뇨병 선별검사
  - Words, 어휘
  - Review, 복습문제

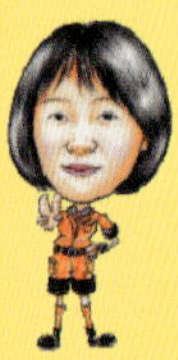

이 책의 녹음 파일은 www.ohgieun.com 에서 무료다운로드 하실 수 있습니다

Oral Glucose Tolerance Test (OGTT)

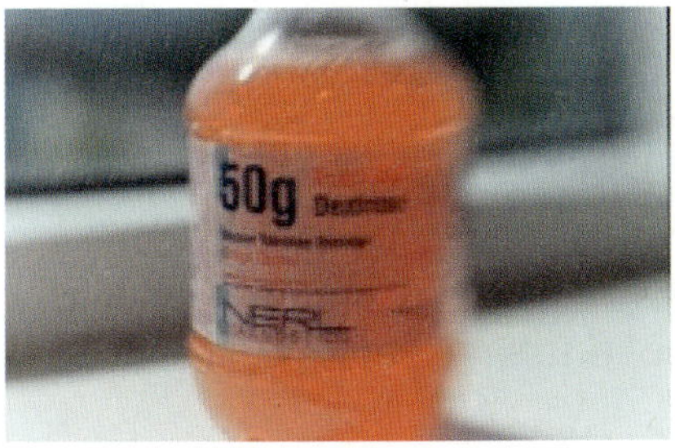

Glucose Tolerance Drink

Glucose tolerance tests are one of the tools used to diagnose diabetes. The most common glucose tolerance test is the oral glucose tolerance test. The oral glucose tolerance test is used to screen pregnant women for gestational diabetes between 24 and 28 weeks of pregnancy. For the test you cannot eat or drink anything after midnight before the test and you cannot eat during the test as well. You will be asked to drink a liquid called glucose tolerance drink containing a certain amount of glucose.

Your blood will be taken before you do this, and again every 30 to 60 minutes after you drink the solution. The test takes up to 3 hours.

Words

oral glucose tolerance test: 경구당부하검사

diabetes/diabetes mellitus: 당뇨병

gestational diabetes: 임신성 당뇨병

glucose tolerance drink: 당부하검사 시약 (포도당)

glucose: 포도당

solution: 시약

Story of My Blood Work

Gestational Diabetes Screening Test

At OB/GYN Clinic

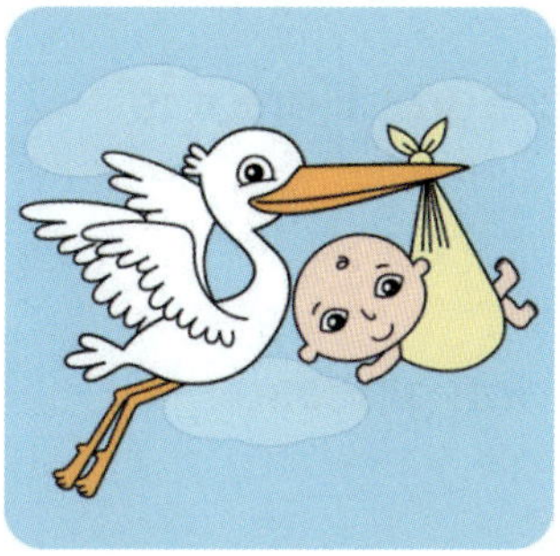

Doctor: I am going to run several tests for you. First, you need to have a oral glucose tolerance test taken.

Patient: I see.

Doctor: For this test, you should fast beforehand.

Patient: Well, how long should I fast?

Doctor: You are required to fast for twelve hours before you have your first blood taken. You will be scheduled for the test early in the day. With a morning appointment you won't be missing two meals by the time you have your blood drawn for the oral glucose tolerance test.

Patient: Thank you for your consideration.

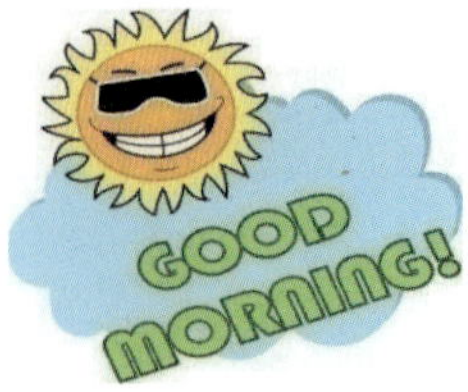

next morning

At the Blood Lab Front Desk

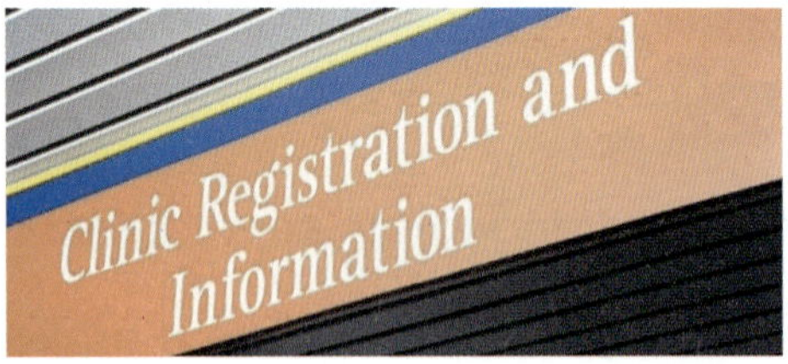

Receptionist: Can I see your blood test slip please?

Patient: Sure. Here it is.

Receptionist: You are scheduled for the oral glucose tolerance test, right?

Patient: That's right. I've been told that I need to do this test on an empty stomach.

Receptionist: That's correct, ma'am. When did you have your last meal?

Patient: I had it at 7:00 p.m. last evening.

Receptionist: Good. Please go to the blood drawing room. Then, you will have your first blood taken.

Patient: I see. Where is the blood drawing room?

Receptionist: It is in the middle of the hallway on this level. It's right next to the waiting area.

Patient: Alright. Thank you.

At the Blood Drawing Room

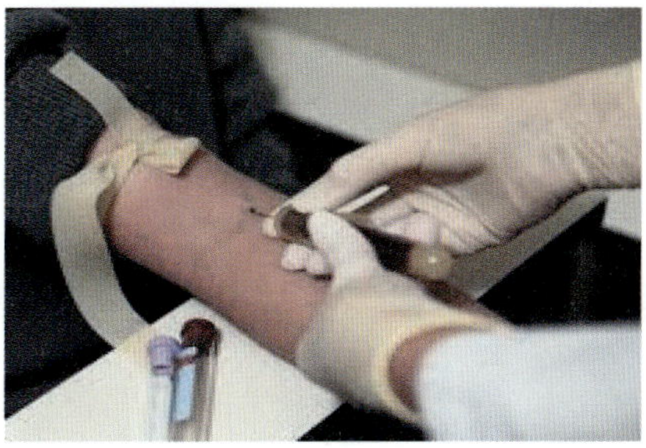

Phlebotomist: Could you state your name and date of birth, please?

Patient: Sunny Anderson and 02/25/72.

Phlebotomist: Alright. Have a seat and sign your name on this paper please.

Patient: Right here?

Phlebotomist: Yes. At the bottom of the paper, please.

Patient: I am finished. Here you are.

Phlebotomist: Thank you. We need to run some tests, so I am going to take a blood sample from you.

Patient: O.K.

Phlebotomist: Please place your arm here. I am going to place this tourniquet on your arm and disinfect the area with alcohol swab. You will feel a little tight.

Patient: I see.

Phlebotomist: Would you please make a fist and squeeze tightly?

Patient: I hope you can find my veins easily.

Phlebotomist: Oh, you have good veins; there should be no problem.

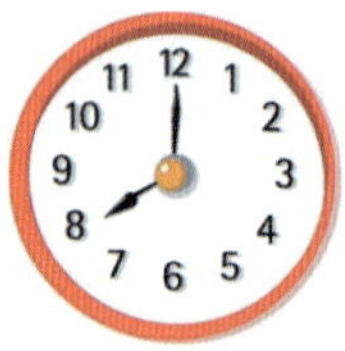

2 minutes later

Phlebotomist: We are all finished now. You can relax your hand now.

Patient: Okay.

Phlebotomist: Please press here for a few minutes and don't rub the puncture mark.

Patient: Alright.

Phlebotomist: If the puncture area keeps bleeding, please let us know immediately.
Patient: I will.

Lab assistant: Now, I will give you orange colored sugary liquid for the next procedure. You need to drink it all.
Patient: Does it make me feel sick or something like that?

Lab assistant: I know the taste is not quite pleasant, but it's not going to make you feel sick. Don't worry about it please. Also, I will give you the oral glucose tolerance test sheet. On the oral glucose tolerance test sheet, you need to note the time when you finish taking this glucose solution.
Patient: I see. I am taking the solution now. It's two o' clock. Let me note the time here.

Lab assistant: Good. You will come back here to have your blood drawn at 2:30, 3:00, and 4:00. I will write the times for you. You should be here 5 minutes before each blood draw.
Patient: I see.

Lab assistant: There is one more thing. You are not allowed to drink water until you finish the test.

Words

gestational diabetes screening test: 임신성 당뇨병 선별검사

OB/GYN: 산부인과

run several tests: 몇 가지 검사를 하다.

oral glucose tolerance test: 경구당부하검사

fast: 금식

beforehand: ~전에

consideration: 배려

on an empty stomach: 공복에

blood drawing room: 채혈실

in the middle of the hallway: 복도의 중간에

at the bottom of: ~의 하단에

disinfect: 소독하다.

make a fist: 주먹을 쥐세요.

sugary liquid: 포도당 시약(설명시 “설탕물보다 더 달다”)

note the time: 시간을 기록하세요.

solution: 시약

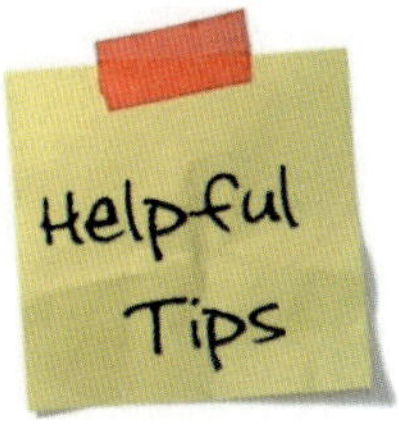

OGTT Results: 경구당부하검사 결과수치

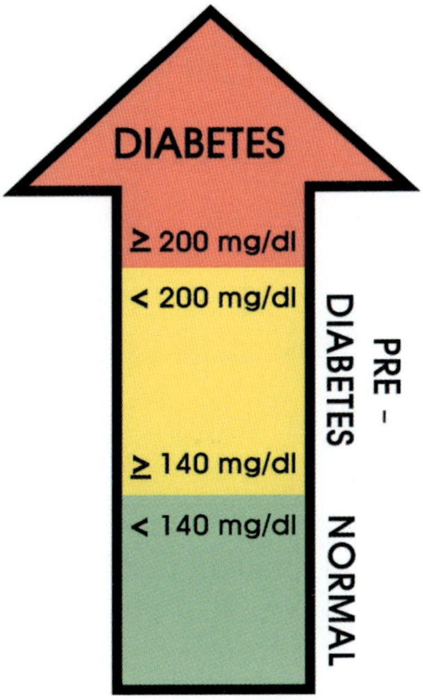

www. hcrefund.com

Review 각각의 구문을 영작하세요.
정답은 전 페이지의 Dialogue를 참고하세요.

At OB/GYN Clinic

Doctor: 몇 가지 검사를 하겠습니다. ....

먼저, 경구당부하검사를 하겠습니다. ....

....

Patient: I see.

Doctor: 이 검사를 받기 위해서는, 검사 전에 금식이 필요합니다.

....

Patient: Well, how long should I fast?

Doctor: 첫 번째 채혈을 하기 12시간 전부터 금식을 하셔야 합니다. ....

검사는 아침 이른 시간으로 예약이 될 것입니다. ....

....

이른 아침에 경구당부하검사를 받게 되면, 검사를 위한 채혈이 시행될 때까지 두 끼를 거르지 않으셔도 됩니다. ....

....

Patient: Thank you for your consideration.

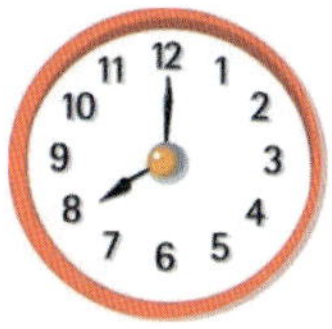

next morning

At the Blood Lab Front Desk

Receptionist: 혈액검사용지를 볼 수 있을까요?

Patient: Sure. Here it is.

Receptionist: 경구당부하검사를 하기로 예약되셨군요, 그렇지요?

Patient: That's right.

공복에 하는 검사라고 들었습니다.

Receptionist: That's correct, ma'am.

언제 마지막으로 식사를 하셨습니까?

Patient: I had it at 7:00 p.m. last evening.

Receptionist: 잘 하셨습니다. 채혈실로 가셔서 첫 번째 채혈을 하십시오.

Patient: I see. Where is the blood drawing room?

Receptionist: 같은 층 복도 중간에 있습니다. 대기실 바로 옆에 있습니다. ....

....

Patient: Alright. Thank you.

At the Blood Drawing Room

Phlebotomist: Could you state your name and date of birth, please?

Patient: Sunny Anderson and 02/25/72.

Phlebotomist: 알겠습니다. 앉으시고 이 용지에 서명하세요. ......

....

Patient: Right here?

Phlebotomist: 예. 용지 하단에요. ....

....

Patient: I am finished. Here you are.

Phlebotomist: Thank you.

몇 가지 검사를 하기 위해 채혈을 하겠습니다. ....

....

Patient: O.K.

Phlebotomist: 여기에 팔을 올려놓으세요. ....

....

토니켓을 팔뚝에 감고 채혈할 부위를 알코올 솜으로 소독하겠습니다. ....

....

조금 조이는 듯한 느낌이 들 것입니다. ....

Patient: I see.

Phlebotomist: 주먹을 꽉 쥐세요. ....

Patient: I hope you can find my veins easily.

Phlebotomist: 핏줄(정맥)이 잘 보여요. 걱정하지 않으셔도 되요.

....

2 minutes later

Phlebotomist: We are all finished now.

이제 주먹을 펴도 됩니다. ....

Patient: Okay.

Phlebotomist: 잠시 동안 누르고 계세요. 채혈한 부위를 문지르지 마세요. ....

....

Patient: Alright.

Phlebotomist: 만일 채혈한 부위에서 피가 멈추지 않는다면, 즉시 알려주세요. ....

....

Patient: I will.

Lab assistant: 이제 다음 검사를 위해 주황색의 설탕물처럼 단 포도당 시약을 드리겠습니다. 다 마셔야 합니다. ....

....

Patient: Does it make me feel sick or something like that?

Lab assistant: 맛은 좋지는 않지만, 속을 이상하게 하지는 않습니다. ....

....

걱정 마세요. 또한, 경구당부하검사용지도 드리겠습니다. ....

....

포도당 시약을 다 마신 후 그 시간을 경구당부하검사용지에 기록하세요. ....

....

Patient: I see. I am taking the solution now. It's two o' clock. Let me note the time here.

Lab assistant: 잘하셨습니다. 이곳으로 2:30, 3:00, 그리고 4:00에 다시 와서 채혈을 하세요. ....

....

제가 시간을 적어드리겠습니다. ....

....

매번 채혈하기 5분전에는 도착해야 합니다. ....

....

Patient: I see.

Lab assistant: There is one more thing.

이 검사가 다 끝날 때까지 물을 마시면 안 됩니다. ....

....

6. Lab Results
검사결과

- **Discussing the Lab Results, 검사결과상담**
    - Dialogue: Abnormal Test Results, 대화: 이상소견을 보이는 검사결과
    - Words, 어휘
    - Review, 복습
- **Discussing the Lab Results, 검사결과상담**
    - Dialogue: Normal Test Results, 대화: 정상인 검사결과
    - Words, 어휘
    - Review, 복습
- **Word Review, 어휘복습**

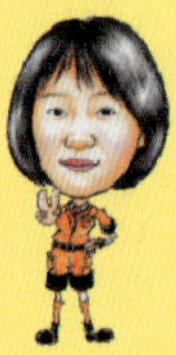

이 책의 녹음 파일은 www.ohgieun.com 에서
무료다운로드 하실 수 있습니다

Discussing the Lab Results

Abnormal Test Results

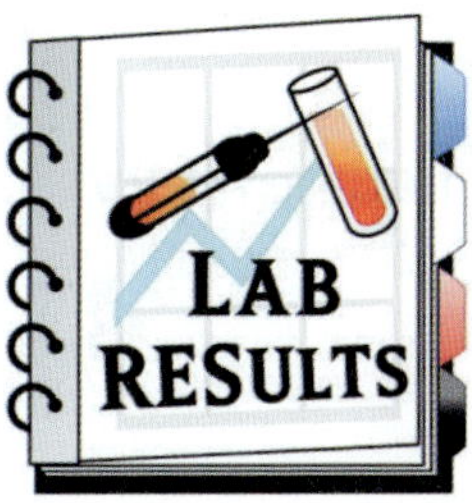

Patient: Hello. I am Mark Anderson. I have an appointment with Dr. Kim regarding my lab results.

Doctor's office Assistant: Alright. Let me check first.

Mr. Anderson: Okay.

Doctor's office Assistant: Mr. Anderson. Please have a seat and a nurse will call you soon.

Nurse: Mr. Anderson. Come in please.

Mr. Anderson: Thank you.

Dr. Kim: Hello, Mr. Anderson. How was your trip to the hospital today?

Mr. Anderson: It wasn't that bad.

Dr. Kim: Good to hear that. By the way, how do you feel now? Are you still feeling nauseous?

Mr. Anderson: Not any more. Since I took the medicines that you prescribed for me, I haven't felt any discomforts in my stomach.

Dr. Kim: Great. Um, your test results have come in, but I'd like to run more tests.

Mr. Anderson: Does this mean that you have bad news for me?

Dr. Kim: No. Sometimes the test results aren't clear, so we need to run more tests to get a clearer picture.

Mr. Anderson: Can we talk about it right now?

Dr. Kim: I would if I knew anything for sure, but I want to take a second look.

Mr. Anderson: I know for sure that something is wrong!

Dr. Kim: We'll know more in a few days. Don't worry about a thing; we are just taking a second look.

Mr. Anderson: I do hope so.

Words

abnormal test results: 이상소견을 보이는 검사결과

regarding my lab results: 제 검사결과에 대해

nauseous: 오심(메스꺼움)

prescribe: (약을)처방하다

run more tests: 추가검사를 하다

clear: 명확한

to get a clearer picture: 정확한 결과를 얻기 위해

I know for sure~: ~에 대하여 확신하다

in a few days: 며칠 후에

take a second look: 재검 하다, 재차 확인하다

Review 각각의 구문을 영작하세요.

정답은 전 페이지의 Dialogue를 참고하세요.

Patient: Hello. I am Mark Anderson.

검사결과를 알기 위해 Dr. Kim 과 예약을 했습니다. ....

....

Doctor's office Assistant: Alright. Let me check first.

Mr. Anderson: Okay.

Doctor's office Assistant: 앤더슨 선생님. 앉아계시면

담당간호사선생님이 호명 할 것입니다. ....

....

Nurse: 앤더슨 선생님. 들어오세요. ....

Mr. Anderson: Thank you.

Dr. Kim: 안녕하세요, 앤더슨 선생님. 병원에 오시는데 별 문제는

없었나요? ....

....

Mr. Anderson: It wasn't that bad.

Dr. Kim: Good to hear that. By the way, how do you feel now? Are you still feeling nauseous?

Mr. Anderson: Not any more. Since I took the medicines that you prescribed for me, I haven't felt any discomforts in my stomach.

Dr. Kim: 다행이군요. 음. 선생님의 검사 결과를 받았습니다. 그런데 추가 검사를 하려고 합니다. ....

....

Mr. Anderson: 결과가 안 좋다는 것인가요?

....

Dr. Kim: 아닙니다. 종종 검사결과가 명확하지 않아서 더 정확한 결과를 얻기 위해 몇 가지 추가검사가 필요합니다. ....

....

Mr. Anderson: 검사결과에 대해 지금 말씀해 주시겠습니까?

....

Dr. Kim: 확실하다면 말씀을 드리겠지만, 재검이 필요합니다.

....

Mr. Anderson: I know for sure that something is wrong!

Dr. Kim: 며칠 후면 알게 될 것입니다. 걱정 마세요. 단지 재검하는 것입니다. ....

....

Mr. Anderson: I do hope so.

Discussing the Test Results

Normal Test Results

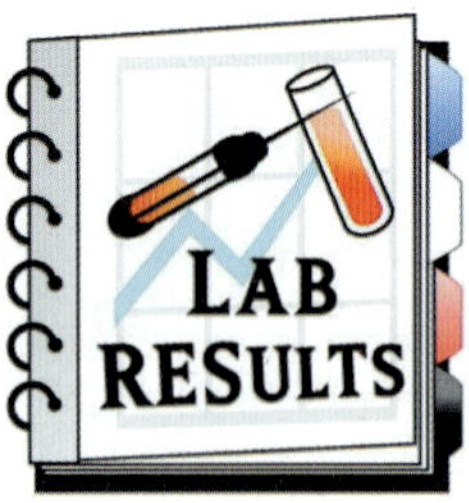

Patient: I am Sunny Anderson. I have an appointment to see the doctor regarding my blood work results.

Doctor's office Assistant: Alright. Could you wait for a minute please?

Ms. Anderson: Sure.

Doctor's office Assistant: Ms. Anderson. Your doctor is waiting for you.

Ms. Anderson: Thank you.

Doctor: Hello, Ms. Anderson. How are you feeling today?

Ms. Anderson: A bit better.

Doctor: That's good to hear. Your test results came in this morning.

Ms. Anderson: Is it good news or bad news?

Doctor: It's good news. I didn't see anything out of ordinary from your lab results. Your blood test came back negative.

Ms. Anderson: Are you saying that there weren't any problems?

Doctor: That's right. There are no major problems.

Ms. Anderson: Thank you for the good news, doctor.

Doctor: No problem.

Words

out of ordinary: 비정상적인

lab results: 검사결과

negative: 질병이 없는

major problem: 심각한 질환, 문제

Review 각각의 구문을 영작하세요.
정답은 전 페이지의 Dialogue를 참고하세요.

Patient: I am Sunny Anderson.

혈액검사결과를 알기 위해 예약을 했습니다. ....

....

Doctor's office Assistant: 알겠습니다. 잠시만 기다려 주시겠습니까? ....

....

Ms. Anderson: Sure.

Doctor's office Assistant: 앤더슨 선생님. 주치의가 기다리고 있습니다. ....

Ms. Anderson: Thank you.

Doctor: Hello, Ms. Anderson. How are you feeling today?

Ms. Anderson: A bit better.

Doctor: That's good to hear.

오늘 아침에 검사결과를 받았습니다. ....

....

Ms. Anderson: 좋은 결과인가요 아니면 안 좋은 결과인가요?

Doctor: 좋은 결과입니다. 검사결과에서 비정상적인 소견은 없습니다.

혈액검사결과는 정상입니다.

Ms. Anderson: 아무런 문제가 없다는 뜻인가요?

Doctor: 맞습니다. 심각한 질환이 없습니다.

Ms. Anderson: 좋은 검사결과를 알려줘서 감사합니다.

Doctor: No problem.

Word Review: 위의 단어들을 복습하는 공간입니다.
정답은 Key Words를 참고하세요.

뜻: In English

혈액검사: ....

채혈사: ....

채혈실: ....

혈액검사실: ....

혈액검체 용기: ....

정맥채혈: ....

토니켓/압박고무줄: ....

주먹을 쥐다/주먹을 꽉 쥐다: ....

손을 펴세요: ....

따끔함: ....

손가락 천자 혈액검사: ....

영아 발뒤꿈치 천자 혈액검사: ....

검사용지: ....

혈액검사용지: ....

7. Urinalysis

소변검사

- **Key Words, 주요어휘**
  - QUIZ: 내 단어장 점검하기
  - Drill: Word Search Puzzle, 연습문제: 어휘퍼즐
- **Reading Material: What is Midstream Urine Collection Method?, 중간뇨 검체 채취방법이란?**
  - Words, 어휘
- **Key Expressions for Urinalysis, 소변검사관련 주요구문**
  - Words, 어휘
  - Drill, 연습문제

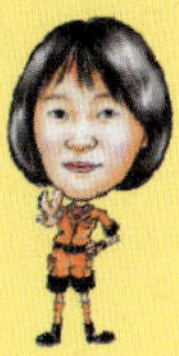

이 책의 녹음 파일은 www.ohgieun.com 에서 무료다운로드 하실 수 있습니다

Key Words

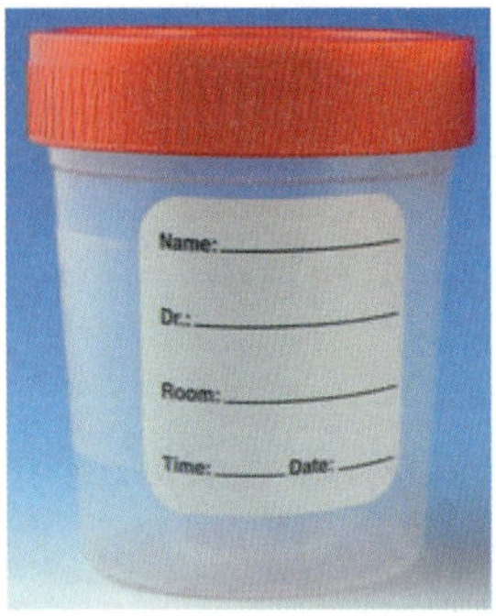

Clean catch/Clean catch urine collection method/Midstream urine collection method: 중간뇨 검체 채취방법

Midstream voided urine: 중간뇨

First flow of urine: 처음 소변

Void: 소변을 누다

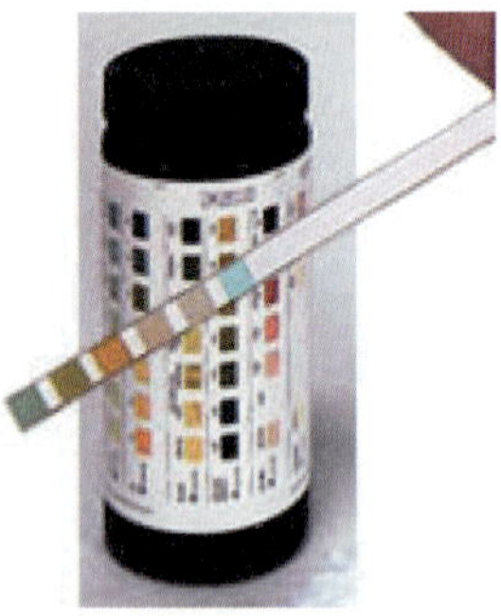

Urine dipstick test: 소변시험지검사법

Urine sample container: 소변검체 용기

Urine collection cup: 소변컵

Random urinalysis: 일반 소변검사

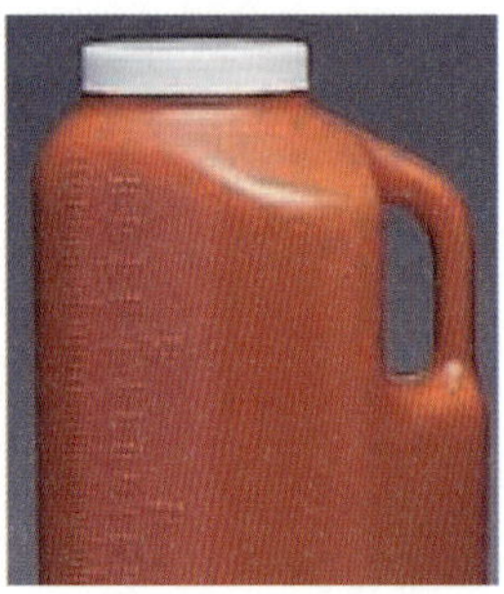

Urine culture: 소변 배양

24-Hour urine sample: 24시간 소변 검체

24-Hour urine collection bottle/bag: 24시간 소변 검체 채취 용기/백

QUIZ: 내 단어장 점검하기 !!

아래 단어를 읽고 알맞은 뜻을 적어보세요..

Clean catch/Clean catch urine collection method: ....

....

Void: ....

First flow of urine: ....

Midstream voided urine: ....

Urine sample container: ....

Urine collection cup: ....

Urine dipstick test: ....

Random urinalysis: ....

Urine culture: ....

24-Hour urine sample: ....

24-Hour urine collection bottle/bag: ....

Drill: 아래의 단어를 ***Word Search Puzzle***에서 찾아보세요.

```
P K P X V R R G G D T U Y D W V J U I V B O
G V P I B H B X V C O R U Q H B N E O V G D
T L R A N D O M   U R I N A L Y S I S X K Q
O D U L F W C N H P F N K A F M D D J O V O
W D K K J V F R S J Q E F W P N F S H X K C
U A E B J C P X S S T   S O Q X D R C G T S
W A U K J L Y C C T G S L E I U P E S D Q J
B L B I J C U A S X C A B F I U X H W Q K O
T V A R G V L P K R S M L X R L H K K Q Y U
K P N P M Q R E G M B P C I A F L N I Q D M
N S N R Y H C C A R D L N C P O C N H R L E
C F V S R K N X J N I E R P Y I X Y C X L U
Q I Y N X Y O E Y T     U P U K L F D M W U
T F V Y U B Y U E C L C H L D R P L T E T R
H G W G V U S C U H V O A G M K N W Q O K E
R K D U R W R L D N F N V T N P G O F L T B
S G S I G R T H R C X T W Y C Y B J E U J U
Y R R S J U U X T L L A J K T H H P K U V I
H O W U R V R K U W Y I T F J N W X L Q O Y
G Y A E Y D N H C L Q N X Y W O J W L Y G G
R D H F C B E P E Y M E L E Y X T O L G T R
Q K N K J A I C J E N R V Y W A G Q Q V Q N
```

소변을 누다, 일반 소변검사, 소변 배양,

소변검체 용기, 중간뇨 검체 채취방법

Reading Material

What is Midstream Urine Collection Method?

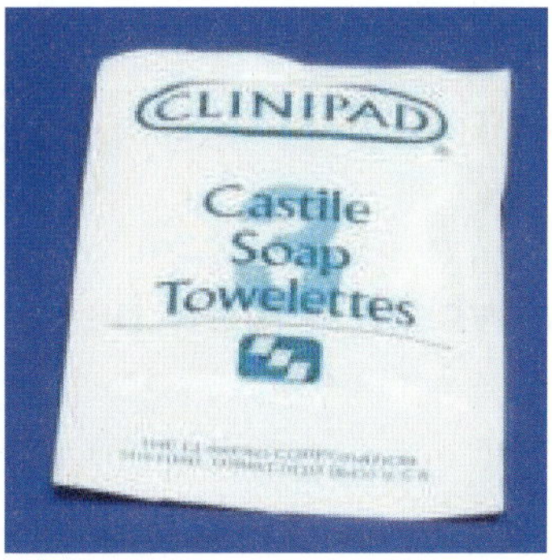

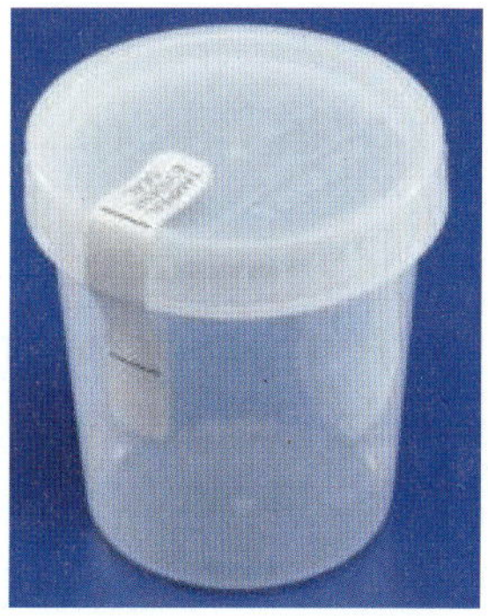

The midstream urine collection method is used to prevent bacteria from genital area from getting into a urine sample. This method can be used for a routine urinalysis, a urine culture, or other urine tests that require pure urine for accurate results.

Words

midstream urine collection method: 중간뇨 검체 채취방법

genital area: 생식기부위

routine urinalysis: 일반 소변검사

urine culture: 소변 배양

Key Expressions for Urinalysis

About Urinalysis

Q1. What is this test for?/What kind of test is this?

A1. Your doctor wants to know whether you have a protein in the urine.

A1-1. Your doctor thinks you have a UTI, so she wants to test your urine.

A1-2. Your doctor ordered 24-hour urine test to see how well your kidneys are working.

About Urine Sample Container

Q2. Why are you handing me a plastic container?/ What do I do with the cup?

A2. Your doctor wants to do a urine test, so this cup is for colleting urine specimen.

A2-1. This big bottle/bag is for a 24-hour urine specimen.

About the Procedure

Q3. How am I supposed to do that?/Am I supposed to urinate into the cup?

A3. After you have urinated a little into the toilet like you normally would, stop the flow and urinate into the urine collection cup until it is about half full.

A3-1. You must collect all urine that you pass in a 24-hour period for this test.

About the Container After Collecting Urine

Q4. What am I suppose to do with the urine cup when I am done?/When I finish, what should I do then?

A4. You need to put the lid tightly on the urine collection cup and leave it in the urine sample tray in the restroom and walk away.

A4-1. You need to leave the urine collection cup on the shelf in the restroom, and the lab tech will get it for you.

About the Test Results

Q5. How long will it take to get the results?/Will I know the results right away?/When will I know the results?

A5. When we send your doctor the results, he/she will discuss it with you.

A5-1. You'll know more in a few days.

A5-3. Your test results have come in.

A5-4. Your urine test came back negative.

Words

protein in the urine/proteinuria: 단백뇨

UTI: Urinary Tract Infection: 요로감염

kidney: 신장

stop the flow: 소변을 참다

urine collection cup: 소변컵

about half full: 대략 반(1/2)정도

lid: 마개, 뚜껑

urine sample tray: 소변 검체를 담는 트레이

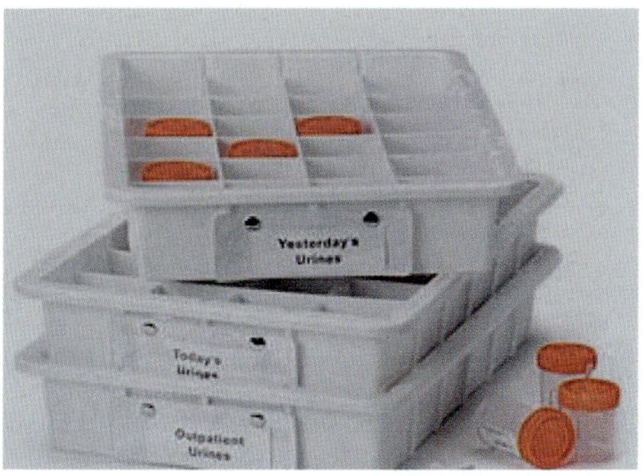

on the shelf: 선반 위에

lab tech: 검사원

Drill: Q1-Q24를 영작하세요.

정답은 전 페이지의 Key Expressions for Urinalysis를 참고하세요.

Q1. 이것은 무슨 검사인가요? ....

Q2. 이 검사는 어떤 검사인가요? ....

Q3. 환자의 담당의사는 환자가 단백뇨가 나오는지 확인하려고 합니다.

....

Q4. 담당의사는 환자가 요로감염이 있다고 생각합니다, 그래서 소변 검사를 하려고 합니다. ....

....

Q5. 환자의 담당의사가 신장의 기능이 정상인지를 알기 위해 24시간 소변검사를 지시했습니다. ....

....

Q6. 왜 플라스틱 용기를 주는 거지요? ....

....

Q7. 이 컵은 어디에 사용하는 것인가요?..

....

Q8. 환자의 담당의사가 소변검사를 원합니다, 그래서 이것은 소변 검체를 담을 컵입니다. ....

Q9. 이 큰 병/주머니는 24시간 소변검체 용기입니다. ....

....

Q10. 어떻게 해야 하는 것인가요? ....

Q11. 이 컵에 소변을 받아야 하나요? ....

Q12. 평상시처럼 변기에 소변을 조금 본 후 멈추고 소변컵에 절반가량 차도록 소변을 보세요. ....

....

Q13. 이 검사를 위해 24시간 동안 소변을 모아야 합니다. ....

....

Q14. 소변을 다 받은 후에 소변컵을 어떻게 해야 하나요?

....

Q15. 마치고 나면, 어떻게 해야 하나요? ....

....

Q16. 소변컵의 마개를 꼭 막고 화장실에 있는 소변 검체를 담는 트레이에 놓고 나오시면 됩니다. ....

....

Q17. 화장실의 선반 위에 소변컵을 놓으면 검사원이 수거할 것입니다. ....

Q18. 검사결과를 알려면 얼마나 걸리나요? ....

....

Q19. 검사결과를 즉시 알 수 있을까요? ....

....

Q20. 언제 검사결과를 알 수 있을까요? ....

....

Q21. 담당의사에게 검사결과가 전달되면, 결과를 환자와 상의할 것 입니다. ....

Q22. 며칠 후에 자세히 알게 될 것입니다. ....
....

Q23. 검사 결과가 나왔습니다. ....

Q24. 소변검사에서 이상소견이 발견되지 않았습니다. ....
....

8. Urine Dipstick Test
시험지 검사법

- **Urine Dipstick Test, 시험지 검사법**
  - Words, 어휘
- **Story of My Urinalysis, 나의 소변검사 이야기**
  - Dialogue: Dipstick Urine Test for Proteinuria, 대화구문: 단백뇨검사
  - Words, 어휘
  - Review, 복습

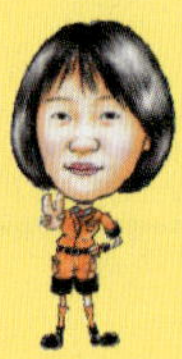

이 책의 녹음 파일은 www.ohgieun.com 에서 무료다운로드 하실 수 있습니다

Urine Dipstick Test

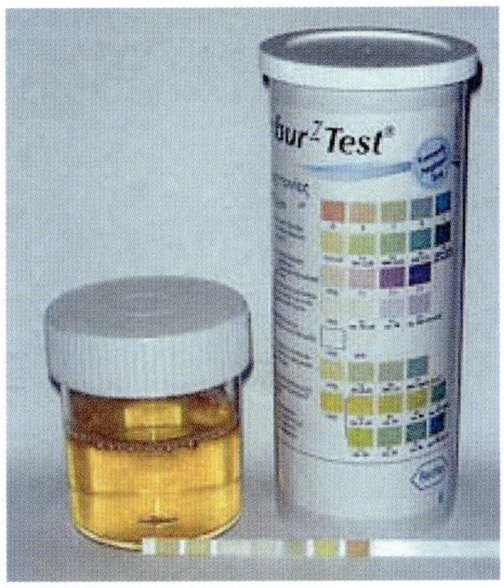

A urine dipstick test is often done as part of an overall urinalysis, but it can also be done on its own, depending on the doctor's concerns. Once a urine sample is collected, a nurse or technician will place a specially treated chemical strip (dipstick) into your urine. Patches on the dipstick will change color to indicate the presence of such things as white blood cells, protein, or glucose.

Words

urine dipstick test: 시험지 검사법

chemical strip (dipstick): 검사용 시험지

Story of My Urinalysis

Dipstick Urine Test For Proteinuria

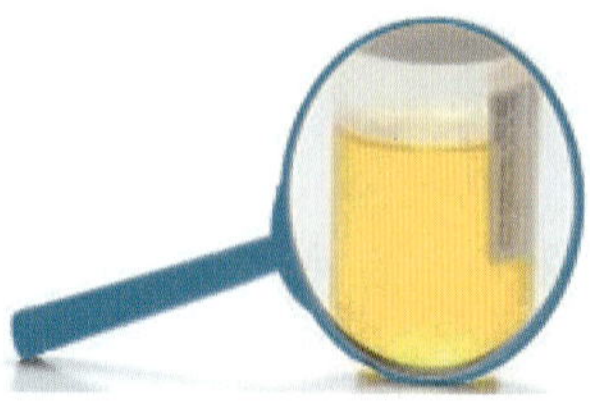

Patient: I am here for a urine test.

Lab Assistant: Alright. Let me verify a couple of things first. What is your name and date of birth, please?

Patient: Linda Soto and 06/12/81.

Lab Assistant: Your doctor wants to know if you have a protein in the urine. Here is your urine collection cup and towelette.

Patient: What's this towelette for?

Lab Assistant: That's for your midstream urine specimen. Since your doctor ordered a protein urine test, we need your midstream urine specimen.

Patient: How am I supposed to collect midstream urine specimen?

Lab Assistant: I will give you instructions for that. First of all, you need to wash your hands and you shouldn't touch the inside of urine collection cup.

Patient: I see.

Lab Assistant: Before collecting urine specimen, you should wipe your urethral area gently with the towelette from front to back in one stroke and discard it. Repeat it for twice. Do I make myself clear?

Patient: Yes.

Lab Assistant: After that you will remove the lid of the urine collection cup and urinate small amount into the toilet first, not into the urine collection cup.

Patient: You mean I discard the first flow of urine, right?

Lab Assistant: That's correct. Then collect the urine to about one third of the urine collection cup and finish voiding into the toilet. When you are done, you need to replace the cap tightly on the urine collection cup. Are you with me so far?

Patient: Yes, I am. Then what am I supposed to do with the cup when I finish?

Lab Assistant: You can leave the urine collection cup in the urine sample tray in the restroom and walk away.

Patient: Okay. Will I know the test results today?

Lab Assistant: Yes, you will.

Words

urine: 소변

towelette: 물수건

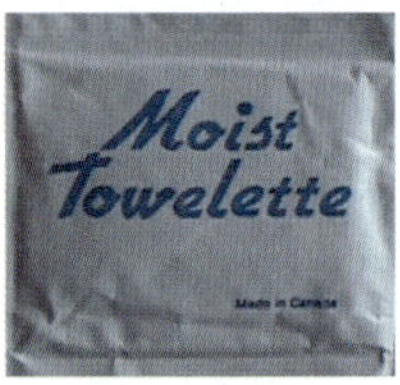

urethral area: 요도부위

one stroke: 한 번에

discard: 버리다

urinate: 배뇨하다

first flow of urine: 첫 소변, 처음 소변

urine sample tray: 소변 검체를 담는 트레이

Review 각각의 구문을 영작하세요.
정답은 전 페이지의 Dialogue를 참고하세요.

Patient: 소변검사를 받으러 왔습니다. ....

....

Lab Assistant: Alright. Let me verify a couple of things first. What is your name and date of birth, please?

Patient: Linda Soto and 06/12/81.

Lab Assistant: 환자의 담당의사는 환자가 단백뇨가 나오는지 확인하려고 합니다. ....

....

Here is your urine collection cup and towelette.

Patient: What's this towelette for?

Lab Assistant: 그것은 중간뇨 검체에 사용됩니다. ....

....

환자의 주치의가 단백뇨 검사를 지시했기 때문에 중간뇨 검체가 필요합니다. ....

....

Patient: 중간뇨를 어떻게 받아와야 하나요? ....

....

Lab Assistant: I will give you instructions for that.

우선 손을 씻으세요. 그리고 소변컵의 안쪽을 만지지 마세요. ....

....

Patient: I see.

Lab Assistant: 소변 검체를 채집하기 전에 요도부위를 물티슈로 앞쪽에서 뒤로 한번에 닦고 물티슈를 버리세요. ....

....

Repeat it for twice. Do I make myself clear?

Patient: Yes.

Lab Assistant: 그런 다음 소변컵의 마개를 연 후에 소량의 소변을 소변컵이 아닌 변기에 보세요. ....

....

Patient: You mean I discard the first flow of urine, right?

Lab Assistant: That's correct.

그런 다음에 소변컵에 1/3가량 소변을 보세요. 그리고 나머지 소변은 변기에 보세요. ....

다 끝나면 소변컵의 마개를 꼭 닫으세요. 이해가 되십니까?

....

Patient: Yes, I am. Then what am I supposed to do with the cup when I finish?

Lab Assistant 화장실의 소변 검체를 담는 트레이에 넣고 나오면 됩니다. ....

Patient: Okay. Will I know the test results today?

Lab Assistant: Yes, you will.

9. Random Urinalysis
일반 소변검사

- **Random Urine Specimen, 일반 소변 검체**
  - Words, 어휘
- **Story of My Urinalysis, 나의 소변검사 이야기**
  - Dialogue: Random Urinalysis, 대화구문: 일반 소변검사
  - Words, 어휘
  - Review, 복습

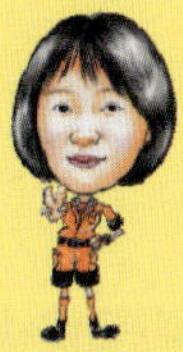

이 책의 녹음 파일은 www.ohgieun.com 에서
무료다운로드 하실 수 있습니다

Random Urine Specimen

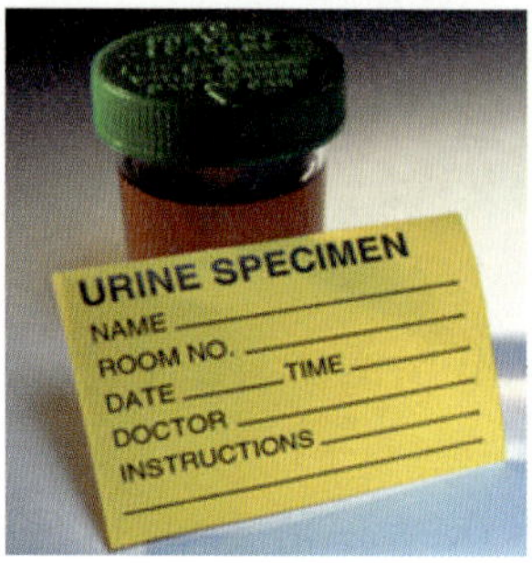

A sample of urine is collected at any time of the day; this type of sample may be used to detect the presence of various substances in the urine at one particular point in the day. Often, no special handling is required with these samples. Other types of urine samples are requested when special types of evaluations are required.

Words

random urine specimen: 일반 소변 검체

at any time of the day: 하루 중 어느 때나

substance: 성분

at one particular point in the day: 하루 중 특정 시간대

no special handling: 특별한 조치 없이

Story of My Urinalysis

Random Urinalysis

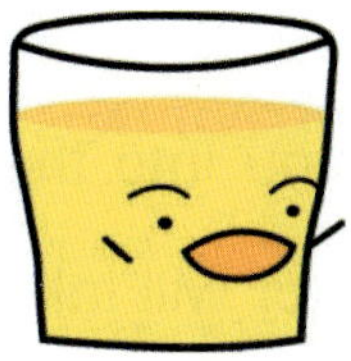

Nurse: Please bring your test slip to the counter.

Patient: Here it is.

Nurse: Could I have your name and date of birth, please?

Patient: Kendra Butler and 04/27/77.

Nurse: Thank you. The test slip says your doctor ordered a urine test. We need your random urine specimen.

Patient: Um. How do I collect random urine sample?

Nurse: I will explain how to collect random urine specimen. First you need to urinate a little into the toilet, stop the flow and urinate into the urine collection cup until it is about half full. Do you understand?

Patient: Yes, I do.

Nurse: Here is a urine collection cup for you. Your name and patient I.D number are on the urine collection cup. When you finish collecting urine sample, please put the cap tightly on the urine collection cup and leave it on the shelf in the restroom. A lab technician will get it for you.

Patient: Alright.

Nurse: Please take the urine collection cup with you into the restroom down this hallway. Your medical coordinator will take you there.

Words

test slip: 검사용지

random urine specimen: 일반 소변 검체

collect: ~을 모으다, 수집하다

stop the flow: 소변을 참다

urine collection cup: 소변컵

about half full: 약 절반 가량

Review 각각의 구문을 영작하세요.
정답은 전 페이지의 Dialogue를 참고하세요.

Nurse: 카운터로 검사용지를 가지고 오세요.

Patient: Here it is.

Nurse: 이름과 생년월일을 말씀해주시겠습니까?

Patient: Kendra Butler and 04/27/77.

Nurse: 감사합니다. 검사용지에 따르면 담당의사선생님이 소변검사를 지시했습니다. 일반 소변 검체가 필요합니다.

Patient: 음. 일반 소변 검체를 어떻게 받아오지요?

Nurse: 일반 소변 검체를 채취하는 방법을 설명해 드리겠습니다.

먼저 변기에 소량의 소변을 보고, 잠시 소변을 멈춘 뒤, 소변컵의 약 절반 가량 채우세요.

Do you understand?

Patient: Yes, I do.

Nurse: 여기 소변컵이 있습니다.

이름과 환자 인식번호가 소변컵에 적혀있습니다.

소변을 다 받은 후에 소변컵의 마개를 꼭 막고 화장실의 선반 위에 소변컵을 놓으세요.

검사원이 수거할 것입니다.

Patient: Alright.

Nurse: 소변컵을 가지고 복도를 따라가 화장실로 가세요.

의료코디네이터가 그 곳으로 안내할 것입니다.

10. 24-hour Urinalysis
24시간 소변검사

- **24-hour Urine Specimen Collection, 24시간 소변 검체 채취**
  - Words, 어휘
- **Instructions for 24-hour Urine Collection, 24시간 소변 채취에 관한 지시사항**
  - Words, 어휘
- **Story of My Urinalysis, 나의 소변검사 이야기**
  - Dialogue: 24-hour Urinalysis, 대화구문: 24시간 소변검사
  - Words, 어휘
  - Review, 복습
- **Word Review, 어휘복습**

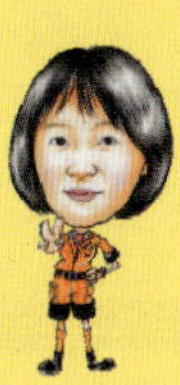

이 책의 녹음 파일은 www.ohgieun.com 에서

무료다운로드 하실 수 있습니다

24-hour Urine Specimen Collection

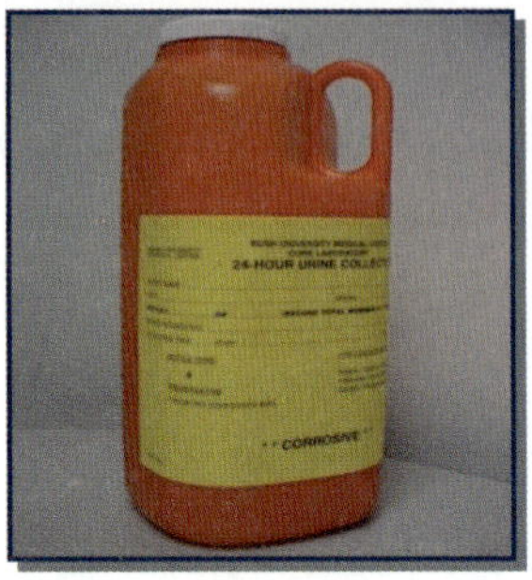

A 24-hour urine collection is when you need to save all the urine you pass in a 24-hour period. This may be needed to measure the amount of certain chemicals your kidneys clean from your body. Some chemicals are cleaned in different amounts during the day and night. With the 24-hour urine the chemical in question can be measured correctly. Another reason to collect your urine for 24 hours may be to see if too little or too much urine is produced.

Words

save: ~을 모으다

pass: 배출하다

certain chemicals: 특정한 성분

clean: 걸러내다

the chemical in question: 검사하려는 성분

Instructions for 24-hour Urine Collection

1. You will be given a 24-hour urine collection bottle. It will need to be kept in the refrigerator or on ice if needed.

2. Always start your 24-hour urine collection in the morning once you begin your collection of urine.

3. Do not save the first urine of the day, but mark this as your start time at the bottom of this sheet.

4. Save all the urine for the next 24 hours in the collection bottle. In order to get the correct results, it is important to save every urine sample. If you forget to save any urine, tell your health care provider. You will need to drink plenty of fluids during this time, 6-8 (8oz.) glasses if possible.

5. The last urine sample should be as close to the starting time as possible and must be saved.

6. Please remember to keep urine in collection bottle in refrigerator or on ice.

7. Bring the bottle(s) to ______________________________

Please fill out the following information:

Patient Name: ____________________________________

Collection Start Date: ________Start Time: ______ AM/PM

Collection Stop Date: ________Stop Time: ______AM/PM

Words

mark: 표기하세요

at the bottom of this sheet: 검사지 아래에

health care provider: 의료진

as close to the starting time as possible: 시작한 시간과 가능한 가까워야 하고

close: 가까운

fill: ~을 기입하세요.

collection: 채취

start date: 시작 날짜

stop date: 종료 날짜

Story of My Urinalysis

24-hour Urinalysis

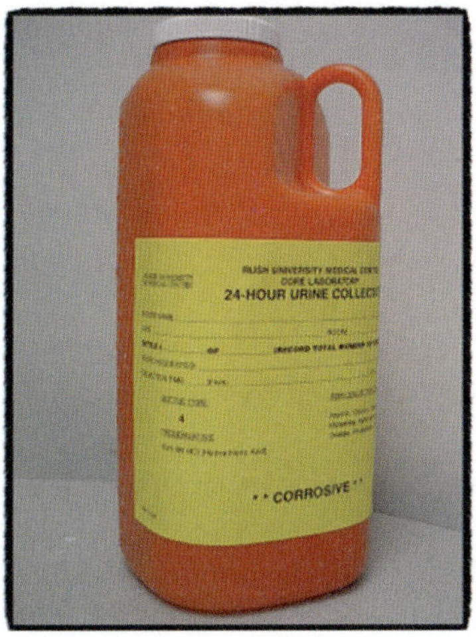

Nurse: Your doctor ordered a 24-hour urine test. I will give you full instructions on how to collect a 24-hour urine sample.

Patient: Alright.

Nurse: First, I'll give you a 24-hour urine collection bottle, urine cup and 24-hour urine collection sheet. You will go home with them. I will write down your name and patient I.D number on the bottle for you.

Patient: Okay.

Nurse: For the next 24-hours, you should save all of your urine and put it into the bottle. If you have a chemical to add, then add it into the 24-hour urine collection bottle first.

Patient: I see.

Nurse: When you begin, you need to empty your bladder in the morning and flush that first urine. After that you will urinate into the urine cup and then pour it into the big bottle.
Patient: You mean I don't save the first urine?

Nurse: That's right. But you need to note the time on the sheet.
Patient: I see.

Nurse: At the end of the 24-hours, you need to urinate one more time and pour the urine into the bottle. Then bring that bottle to the lab the next day with your 24-hour urine collection sheet, please.
Patient: Um. I don't understand the last part. You mean I need to save the urine when the 24-hours is over?

Nurse: That's right. Do you remember the first instruction? You are supposed to flush the first urine instead of saving it but write the time. This is the reason that you need to save the last part of your urine after 24 hours is over.
Patient: Now I've got it.

Nurse: If you miss collecting one or more voids, consult a lab technician in the laboratory for further instructions, please.

Patient: Alright. See you later then.

Words

24-hour urinalysis/24-hour urine test: 24시간 소변검사

full instructions on: ~에 관한 모든 지시사항

24-hour urine collection bottle: 24시간 소변 검체 채취 용기

24-hour urine collection sheet: 24시간 소변 검체 채취 용지

empty your bladder: 소변을 보다

flush: 변기의 물을 내리다

pour: 붓다

note the time: 시간을 기록하다

Review 각각의 구문을 영작하세요.
정답은 전 페이지의 Dialogue를 참고하세요.

Nurse: 의사선생님이 24시간 소변 검사를 지시했습니다.

24시간 소변 검체 채취에 관한 모든 지시사항을 말씀 드리겠습니다. ....

Patient: Alright.

Nurse: 우선 24시간 소변 검체 채취 용기, 소변컵과 24시간 소변 검체 채취 용지를 드리겠습니다. ....

You will go home with them.

환자의 이름과 환자인식번호를 용기에 적겠습니다. ....

Patient: Okay.

Nurse: 다음 24시간 동안 배뇨하는 모든 소변을 검체 용기에 모으세요. ....

만일 소변용기에 첨가할 약품이 있다면 먼저 24시간 소변 검체 채취 용기에 첨가하세요. ....

....

Patient: I see.

Nurse: 검사를 시작할 때, 아침에 소변을 보고 그 첫 소변은 버리세요. ....

....

그 후, 소변컵에 소변을 본 후에 큰 검체 용기에 부으세요. ....

....

Patient: You mean I don't save the first urine?

Nurse: 맞습니다. 하지만 그 시간은 용지에 기록하셔야 합니다.

....

Patient: I see.

Nurse: 24시간이 경과한 후 배뇨한 소변을 한번 더 용기에 모으세요. ....

그리고 다음날 24시간 소변 검체 채취 용기와 24시간 소변 검체 채취 용지도 함께 가지고 검사실로 오세요. ....

....

Patient: Um. I don't understand the last part. You mean I need to save the urine when 24-hours is over?

Nurse: 예, 첫 번째 지시사항을 기억하십니까? ....

....

처음 소변은 모으지 않고 버리되 시간은 기록해야 했지요. ....

....

이것이 24시간이 지난 후의 마지막 부분의 소변을 모아야 하는 이유입니다. ....

....

Patient: Now I've got it.

Nurse: 만일 한 두 번 소변을 모으지 못 했다면, 검사실의 검사원에게 의뢰하여 추가적인 지시사항을 상담 받으세요. ....

....

Patient: Alright. See you later then.

Word Review: 위의 단어들을 복습하는 공간입니다.
정답은 Key Words를 참고하세요.

뜻: In English

중간뇨 검체 채취방법: ____________________

중간뇨: ____________________

처음 소변: ____________________

소변을 누다: ____________________

소변시험지검사법: ____________________

소변검체 용기: ____________________

소변컵: ____________________

일반 소변검사: ____________________

소변 배양: ____________________

24시간 소변 검체: ____________________

24시간 소변 검체 채취 용기/백: ____________________

11. FAQ for the Lab Test
검사에 관련된 자주하는 질문

- **FAQ for the Lab Test, 검사에 관련된 자주하는 질문**

  - Words, 어휘

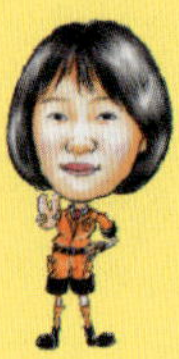

이 책의 녹음 파일은 www.ohgieun.com 에서 무료다운로드 하실 수 있습니다

FAQ for Lab Test

About Lab Test Procedures

Q1. What does fasting mean?

A1. Fasting means no food or drink including water for 6-8 hours before testing. You may take your medications during the fasting interval. Physicians may order patients to fast for certain tests, such as glucose or lipid panels. But not all tests require a patient to fast.

Q2. Can my lab test be ordered anonymously?

A2. Yes. That portion of service is available at our hospital.

A2-1. We currently do not have that capability, although we hope to soon have that portion of our service available to you.

Q3. What do I need to bring when I go to the laboratory?

A3. You need to bring your receipt.

About an Appointment for a Lab Test

Q4. Can I cancel my lab test?

A4. Yes, you can. However, once you have tested, we cannot cancel or refund you the price of labs.

Q5. Do I need an appointment for laboratory tests?

A5. Yes. You need an appointment for the lab tests. Our clinic/hospital is not on walk-in basis, first come first serve.

Q6. What is the appointment process for 3-hour Oral Glucose Tolerance Test (OGTT)?

A6. We will set up an appointment for 3-hour OGTT when you visit your doctor's office. Appointments are set up during weekdays at 9:00 am.

Q7. What do I do if I have any questions?

A7. Please contact us at this number 234-5678 if you have any questions. We will do our best to answer them in a timely manner.

Q8. How long is my lab slip good for?

A8. Once you have received your lab slip, you have certain days to go to the lab center and get your tests done. After this date, the order expires, and you need to get your lab slip from your doctor if you still wish to get your tests done.

About a Lab Facility

Q9. Where is the (Blood) Laboratory located?

A9. The Hospital's Main Laboratory is located on the (first) floor.

Q10. Where can I park?

A10. Patients having laboratory tests can park in any outpatient parking. The closest parking lot to the laboratory is located next to the (Emergency) Department.

Q11. Where do I need to go to have my lab test done?

A11. We have a medical coordinator to take you to the lab. However, if you have any questions about the lab center, please feel free to contact us with any questions.

About Lab Test Results

Q12. When will I get my results?

A12. It depends on the test. If it's not a STAT order, you should receive your results within (5) business days of your lab test, or if it's a STAT order, you should receive your results within an hour or so at the spot.

Q13. How confidential are my results?

A13. We do not share your medical information with any third party without your consent. We observe the Patient's Privacy Policy.

Q14. How will I know what the tests mean?

A14. Most tests will have a range of what is considered normal by that lab's standards. If the test result is out of normal range, a physician will interpret the results for you.

Q15. How reliable are the results?

A15. We routinely provide reliable testing using scientifically proven testing methods. However, there can be issues which affect the accuracy of the sample. For example, some tests require fasting; if you have not fasted, the test will be inaccurate. Another issue may have to do with how the sample itself is processed. If you believe the test results are in error, retesting is recommended.

Q16. Can I get a copy of my results?

A16. Yes, you can. If you request a copy of your results, we can also send the results by mail or fax.

Q17. If I lost my lab results, can I get a copy of mine?

A17. If you have lost your lab results, we can reissue your lab results and send them to you.

About Lab Test Fee

Q18. Do you accept any other forms of payment besides cash?

A18. We do accept credit cards, too.

Q19. Do you accept international medical insurance?

A19. We accept some international medical insurance but not all. Also, if your medical insurance is not under our contract or direct billing arrangement, then you are financially responsible for all expenses and need to pay out-of-pocket.

Q20. Will you file an insurance claim for me?

A20. We do offer that service. However, you may send our invoices to your insurance provider for reimbursement.

Words

anonymously: 익명으로

refund: 환불

at the spot: 그 장소에서

third party: 제 삼자

consent: 동의

observe: 준수하다

Patient's Privacy Policy: 환자의 개인정보 보호 정책

a copy of~: ~의 사본

reissue: 재발급하다

pay out-of-pocket: 자비로 지불하다

file an insurance claim: 보험청구를 하다

invoices: 진료비 관련 청구서

reimbursement: 보상

12. 해석 및 정답

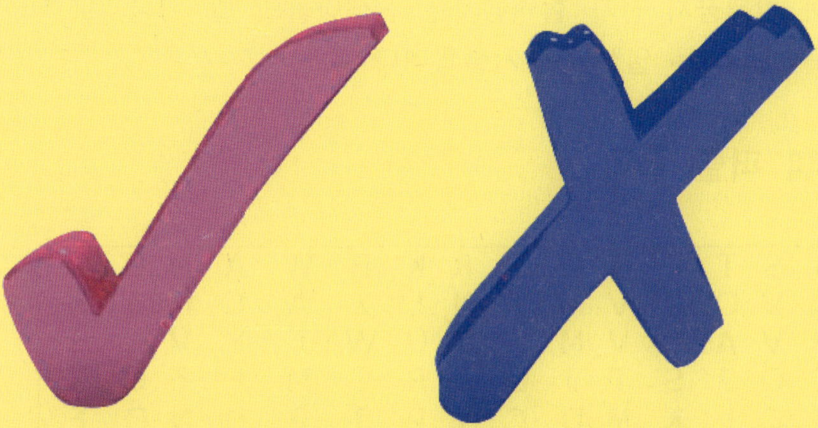

1. Blood Work/Blood Test
혈액검사

Key Words

(채혈을 담당하는 전문인)

토니켓은 채혈사에게 혈관이 더 잘 드러나게 하기 위해 팔뚝에 감겨집니다.

영아 발뒤꿈치 천자 혈액검사는 신생아들의 발 뒤꿈치로부터 혈액을 채취하는 일상적인 시술입니다.

어휘 퍼즐 정답

J	S	T	E	D	O	I	R	K	B	W	A	N	B	O
R	V	O	N	V	M	T	N	L	X	A	C	M	L	X
B	V	A	O	V	M	P	O	U	W	F	Y	V	O	E
P	Q	P	S	T	J	O	G	R	C	M	F	F	O	X
K	C	L	K	M	D	C	Y	P	J	P	D	N	D	F
R	J	X	O		V	A	T	Y	F	D	N	U		W
E	U	O	W	T	O	U	R	N	I	Q	U	E	T	O
B	L	O	O	D	L	A	B	B	T	E	T	S	E	G
O	R	D	P	H	L	E	B	O	T	O	M	I	S	T
K	P	J	O	R	L	L	S	F	T	S	O	G	T	E
D	O	T	G	L	I	E	G	A	B	U	W	S		Q
X	E	I	W	U	I	C	P	R	H	R	P	X	S	T
H	O	F	L	X	C	F	K	C	O	A	I	U	L	U
L	U	S	I	X	N	W	G	X	B	N	V	S	I	D
P	L	P	L	O	K	M	V	T	K	C	J	K	P	B

Phlebotomist	Bloodlab	Tourniquet
Prick	Blood work	Blood test slip

독해구문

나의 혈액검사

질문:

나는 혈액검사를 받아야 합니다. 그런데 3병이나 뽑아야 합니다. 아플까요? 그리고 3병이 많은가요?

답변:

주사바늘이 찌를 거라는 생각이 실제 느끼는 통증보다 더 고통스럽습니다. 일단 주사 바늘이 정맥에 들어가면, 더 이상 아프지 않습니다. 그리고 채혈사나 간호사가 정맥에 주사를 놓는 것이 1초도 안 걸립니다. 됐습니다. 다 끝났습니다.

하하! 절 믿으세요. 세 병은 별 거 아닙니다.

저는 혈액검사에 일가견이 있습니다, 그리고 셀 수 없이 많은 병의 피를 뽑아 봤습니다. 세 병은 별거 아닙니다. 그리고 당신은 검사 후에 아무런 차이를 느끼지 못할 것입니다.

걱정 마세요!

행운을 빌어요!

로리와 함께 하는 미국 문화 엿보기

채혈사란?

채혈사는 다양한 검사와 시술을 하기 위해 환자에게서 채혈을 하는 전문의료인들입니다. 고등학교졸업생 또는 대학재학생들도 직업학교에서 수업을 들으며 채혈하는 방법을 배울 수 있습니다.

채혈에 관하여

채혈이란?

채혈이란 당신의 건강상태를 확인하기 위한 기본검사를 할 수 있도록 혈액검체를 채취하는 방법입니다. 채혈은 약 5-10분 정도 소요됩니다. 채혈 한 부위가 약 하루 정도 아플 수 있으나 채혈 후 당신은 정규식사와 활동을 재게할 수 있습니다.

채혈방법

채혈에는 손가락에서 채혈하는 방법과 정맥에서 채혈하는 두 가지 방법이 있습니다. 손가락채혈은 소량의 혈액을 채취하기 위해 작은 주사바늘을 사용하여 손가락 끝을 찌릅니다. 정맥채혈은 안쪽 팔의 정맥으로부터 채혈하기 위해 주사바늘을 사용합니다.

집에서 준비할 사항

의사선생님의 특별한 지시사항이 없는 한 집에서 준비해야 할 사항은 없습니다. 환자의 주치의가 채혈을 하기 전 일정시간 동안 음식을 섭취하는 것을 금할 수도 있습니다. 주치의가 내린 주의사항을 준수하여 주세요.

채혈전

채혈은 외래진료 시 또는 입원했을 경우 행해집니다. 대부분의 외래진료 시 채혈은 유사한 절차로 진행됩니다. 접수처에서 접수한 후 대기실에서 기다리라는 지시를 받습니다.

채혈 중

환자는 간호사 또는 채혈사와 함께 검사실에 가게 됩니다. 환자는 채혈이 진행되는 동안 의자에 편안히 앉아 있게 됩니다.

채혈 후

간호사 또는 채혈사가 필요한 모든 채혈검체 채집이 끝나고 바늘을 빼면 채혈은 종료된 것입니다. 간호사 또는 채혈사는 정맥채혈 부위를 알코올 솜으로 누른 후 반창고를 붙일 것입니다. 채혈이 끝난 후, 일상적인 활동을 재게 할 수 있습니다. 결과가 나오면, 주치의가 검사결과를 상의할 것입니다.

혈액검사관련 주요구문

Wh-Questions~

1. 혈액검사를 받으러 어디로 가야 하나요?
2. 언제 혈액검사 결과를 알 수 있을까요?/검사 결과를 언제 알 수 있을까요?
3. 이것은 무슨 검사인가요?

Could I/you~
Would I/you~

4. 혈액검사용지를 볼 수 있을까요?
5. 성함이 무엇입니까?
6. 자리에 앉으시고 왼쪽 소매를 올려주시겠습니까?
7. 오른쪽 소매를 올려주시겠습니까?
8. 주먹을 꽉 쥐시겠습니까?
9. 팔을 이 테이블 위에 올려주시겠습니까?
10. 채혈을 할 때 누우시는 것이 더 나을까요?
11. 팔에서 채혈을 하는 동안 움직이지 마세요.

Do you ~?
Did you ~?

12. 바늘에 대한 공포증이 있습니까?

13. 주사공포증이 있습니까?

14. 혈액검사에 관한 질문사항이 있습니까?

15. 검사 전에 먹은 것이 있나요?

Others

16. 아플까요?

17. 검사 전에 제한해야 할 음식이 있습니까?

18. 혈액검사를 받을 때 실신한 적이 있습니까?

19. 혈액검사 결과를 받으려면 보통 얼마나 걸리나요?

20. 이제 주먹을 펴도 됩니다.

21. 다 끝났습니다./이제 다 끝났습니다.

22. 이 압박고무줄/토니켓/고무밴드가 조일 것입니다.

23. 핏줄을 더 잘 드러나게 하기 위해 팔의 윗 부분을 압박 고무줄로 감겠습니다.

24. 핏줄이 더 잘 드러나게 하기 위해 팔뚝에 토니켓을 감겠습니다.

25. 바늘은 비스듬하게 들어가고 혈액은 용기에 담길 것입니다.

2. Cholesterol Test/Lipid Panel Test
콜레스테롤검사/지질검사

바늘 공포증

오늘날, 진단과정뿐만 아니라 예방의학의 관점에서 주사와 혈액검사가 정기적으로 사용되는데 두 가지 모두 바늘이 요구됩니다. 그러나 환자의 약 10%는 바늘 공포증을 겪고 있거나 바늘이나 뾰족한 물건에 심한 공포를 가지고 있습니다. 바늘 공포증이 있는 사람은 주사를 맞는 것 또는 혈액검사를 받는 것에 상당한 공포를 느낀다는 것이 알려졌습니다. 주사공포증은 신체에 직접적으로 느끼는 증상뿐만 아니라 공포로 인하여 진료를 회피하기 때문에 위험할 수 있습니다.

바늘 공포증은 한때는 바늘에 대한 감정적인 반응이며 유년기적 공포라고 여겨졌습니다. 그러나 Dr. James G. Hamilton의 "바늘공포증: 간과된 진단" 이란 한 논문에 의하면 이 공포증은 "어린이들에게만 한정된 것은 아니며, 감정에 의해 발생하는 것도 아니고 일시적인 것도 드문 경우도 아니라고" 언급하였습니다. Dr. Hamilton은 "이것이 흔한 증상이며, 바늘 공포증이 있는 환자들은 치료를 회피하는 경향이 있어 사회적, 법률적 문제 뿐만 아니라 심각한 건강 문제를 일으킬 수 있기 때문에 의사들은 이런 증상에 대해 숙지하고 있어야 한다"고 언급했습니다.
여러 다른 종류의 바늘 공포증이 아래에 예시 되어있습니다.

Belonephobia: 핀과 바늘에 대한 공포증

Trypanophobia: 주사공포증

Aichmophobia: 날카롭고 뾰족한 물건에 대한 공포증

증상

혈압상승(고혈압), 심박동수의 증가(빈맥), 스트레스호르몬 수치상승, 어지럼증 및 의식을 잃을 가능성(혈관미주신경반사)과 같은 신체적 증상들이 심지어 주사를 맞거나 혈액검사를 받을 생각만으로도 나타납니다. 그러므로, 주사가 치료에 필요한 한 부분이라는 것을 환자에게 알려주는 것이 도움이 됩니다.

치료

많은 불안장애들은 약물과 인지활동치료를 병행하며 치료를 하지만, 이런 치료방법은 바늘공포증을 개선하는데 효과가 없는 것 같습니다. 바늘공포증이 있는 사람들에게, 공포증상의 완화에 도움이 되도록 아래의 몇몇 방법들을 의사와 상의하세요.

자세

어지럼증과 의식을 잃는 것이 심각한 문제가 될 수 있으며 이런 증상들은 환자가 주사나 침을 맞는 동안 머리를 낮추고 다리를 올리고 누워있으면 완화될 수가 있습니다. 환자는 안정감을 느낄 때까지 이 자세를 유지해야 하며 천천히 앉거나 일어서야 합니다.

행동전략

주사를 맞기 전에 의사 또는 전문의료인과 당신의 바늘공포증에 대해 상의하세요. 전문의료인은 주사를 놓거나 채혈을 하는데 반드시 숙련되고 능숙해야 합니다. 주사를 맞거나 채혈을 할 때 천천히 깊게 호흡을 하면 신체에 느끼는 다른 증상을 완화 시키는데 도움이 될 것입니다.

콜레스테롤검사/지질검사

콜레스테롤검사/지질검사, 또는 관상동맥질환 고위험군 검사라 불리는 이 테스트는 관상동맥질환의 위험성을 진단하기 위한 검사입니다. 콜레스테롤검사(지질검사)는 **총콜레스테롤, 중성지방, 고지질 지방단백질 콜레스테롤(HDL콜레스테롤) 및 저지질 지방단백질 콜레스테롤(LDL콜레스테롤)의** 수치를 재는 검사 입니다.

총콜레스테롤은 여러 형태의 콜레스테롤의 합계치를 의미합니다. **중성지방은** 신체가 필요할 때 사용하려고 에너지를 저장해 둡니다. 너무 많은 양의 칼로리를 섭취하게 되면 몸은 지방의 형태로 중성지방을 만들어 저장합니다. 만일 몸에 너무 많은 중성지방이 축적 된다면, 혈관은 막히고 질병을 앓게 됩니다.

고밀도 지방단백질 콜레스테롤은 좋은 콜레스테롤이라 불립니다. 고밀도 지방단백질 콜레스테롤은 혈관내의 콜레스테롤을 간으로 운반하여 제거합니다.

저밀도 지방단백질 콜레스테롤은 나쁜 콜레스테롤이라고도 알려져 있습니다. 혈관내에 축적되는 저밀도 지방단백질 콜레스테롤은 혈관을 막히게 하고 심장질환의 위험을 증가시킵니다.

나의 혈액검사 이야기

콜레스테롤검사/지질검사

Nurse: 앤더슨 선생님. 여기 혈액검사용지가 있습니다. 채혈사가 무엇을 해야 하는지 알려줄 것이고 채혈을 할 것입니다.

Ms. Anderson: 알겠습니다. 혈액검사 받으러 어디로 가야 하나요?

Nurse: 환자분의 의료코디네이터가 그곳으로 안내할 것입니다.

Ms. Anderson: 좋군요.

Medical coordinator: 안녕하세요, 앤더슨선생님. 제가 선생님의 의료코디네이터인 에밀리 입니다. 제가 혈액검사실로 안내해 드리겠습니다. 이쪽으로 오세요.

Ms. Anderson: 감사합니다.

Medical coordinator: 별말씀을요.

접수처에서

Medical coordinator: 안녕하세요. 이 환자분의 의사선생님이 혈액검사를 하라고 이곳으로 보냈습니다.

Lab Assistant: 제가 도와드리겠습니다. 환자분의 혈액검사용지를 볼 수 있을까요?

Ms. Anderson: 예. 여기 있습니다.

Lab Assistant: 환자분의 주치의가 콜레스테롤 검사를 처방하셨습니다. 채혈사가 곧 올 것입니다.

Ms. Anderson: 알겠습니다.

Phlebotomist: 안녕하세요. 제가 채혈사입니다. 제가 환자의 팔(전완)에서 채혈을 하겠습니다. 우선 몇 가지 확인을 하겠습니다. 환자분의 성함과 생년월일을 말씀해 주시겠습니까?

Ms. Anderson: 써니 앤더슨이고 1972년 2월 25일 생입니다.

Phlebotomist: 알겠습니다, 앤더슨씨. 바늘에 대한 공포증이 있습니까? 제 말은 혈액검사를 받거나 주사를 맞을 때, 주사바늘에 대한 이해할 수 없을 정도의 공포를 느끼나요?

Ms. Anderson: 그렇지 않습니다.

Phlebotomist: 다행이군요. 앉으셔서 왼쪽 소매를 걷어주시겠습니까?

Ms. Anderson: 이렇게요?

Phlebotomist: 네, 맞습니다.

Ms. Anderson: 긴장이 되요.

Phlebotomist: 핀으로 살짝 찌르는 정도입니다. 그러니 너무 걱정 마세요. 제가 간단하게 진행절차를 설명해 드리겠습니다. 우선 팔의 정맥이 좀더 잘 나타나게 하기 위해 팔의 윗 부분에 토니켓을 감겠습니다. 조금 조이는 듯한 느낌을 받을 것입니다.

Ms. Anderson: 알겠습니다.

Phlebotomist: 그런 후, 채혈하기 위해 팔꿈치의 안쪽 부위를 소독솜으로 닦겠습니다. 제가 주사바늘을 꽂은 후에 혈액을 담기 위해 튜브를 바늘에 연결할 것입니다.

Ms. Anderson: 알겠습니다. 그런데 혈액을 몇 병이나 채취할 것인가요?

Phlebotomist: 튜브 1개를 채혈할 것입니다. 한 가지 더요. 제가 채혈을 할 때 다른 곳을 보고 움직이지 않으면 도움이 되실 것입니다. 준비 되셨나요?

Ms. Anderson: 네.

Phlebotomist: 아픈 느낌이 들 것입니다.

1분 후

Phlebotomist: 채혈이 다 끝났습니다. 필요한 혈액 검체 채취를 끝냈습니다. 이제 채혈한 부위에 거즈를 대겠습니다. 지혈이 되도록 누르시면 됩니다. 하지만 문지르면 안됩니다. 지혈을 돕기 위해 팔을 굽혀주세요. 가시기 전에 다른 질문사항은 없나요?

Ms. Anderson: 음, 채혈부위에 멍도 드나요?

Phlebotomist: 아마도 멍이 들 수도 있고 조금 아플 수도 있습니다.

Ms. Anderson: 알겠습니다. 다른 질문이 있습니다. 결과는 언제 알 수 있을까요?

Phlebotomist: 약 일주일정도 걸립니다. 결과가 환자분의 담당의사에게 전해지면 즉시 알려드리겠습니다.

Ms. Anderson: 감사합니다!

Phlebotomist: 별말씀을요. 내원해주셔서 감사합니다.

3. Complete Blood Count (CBC)Test
전혈구 검사

전혈구 검사

전혈구 검사는 매우 일반적인 검사입니다. 많은 환자들은 그들의 전반적인 건강상태를 점검하기 위해 기본 검사인 전혈구 검사를 합니다. 전혈구 검사는 빈혈, 감염 및 많은 다른 질병을 판별하기 위해 사용됩니다. 이 검사는 적혈구 수, 백혈구 수, 총 헤모글로빈 수 및 혈액의 다른 성분을 검사하는 전반적인 검사입니다.

나의 혈액검사 이야기

긴급검사! 전혈구검사

Lab Assistant: 이름이 무엇입니까?

Patient: 켄 존슨입니다.

Lab Assistant: 존슨 선생님. 혈액검사용지를 보여주시겠습니까?

Mr. Johnson: 여기 있습니다. 무슨 검사인가요?

Lab Assistant: 환자의 담당의사 선생님이 백혈구수치를 보려고 전혈구 검사를 지시했습니다.

Mr. Johnson: 백혈구 수치가 제 담당의사선생님에게 무엇을 알려주는데요?

Lab Assistant: 만일 백혈구 수치가 올라가면 염증이 있다는 것을 말합니다.

Mr. Johnson: 알겠습니다.

Lab Assistant: 여기에 앉으시고 이 서류의 하단에 서명해 주세요.

Mr. Johnson: 알겠습니다.

Lab Assistant: 에밀리, 환자가 있습니다. 환자의 담당의사가 긴급검사로 지시를 내렸습니다. 이 환자의 혈액검사를 급히 해야 합니다. 지금 바로 이 환자의 채혈을 해 주시겠습니까?

Emily (Phlebotomist): 물론이죠. 즉시 하겠습니다.

Lab Assistant: 정말이지 빠르게 도와주셔서 고맙습니다.

Emily (Phlebotomist): 별말씀을요.

Emily (Phlebotomist): 안녕하세요, 제가 채혈사 입니다. 우선 이름과 생년월일을 말씀해 주시겠습니까?

Mr. Johnson: 켄 존슨 이고 1970년 5월 30일생입니다.

Emily (Phlebotomist): 감사합니다. 존슨 선생님. 팔에서 채혈을 하겠습니다. 오른쪽 소매를 걷어주세요.

Mr. Johnson: 나는 오른손잡이입니다, 그래서 항상 왼쪽 팔에서 채혈을 했습니다. 오른팔 대신에 왼쪽 팔에서 채혈을 해주시겠습니까?

Emily (Phlebotomist): 그럼요. 물론이지요. 또 다른 사항은요?

Mr. Johnson: 없습니다.

Emily (Phlebotomist): 그러면, 왼쪽 소매를 걷어주시겠습니까?

Mr. Johnson: 알겠습니다.

Emily (Phlebotomist): 팔을 쭉 펴주세요. 상완을 토니켓으로 묶고 알코올 솜으로 팔을 소독하겠습니다.

Mr. Johnson: 알겠습니다.

Emily (Phlebotomist): 주먹을 세 번 꽉 쥐세요 그리고 마지막 번에서 주먹을 꼭 쥔 채로 계세요.

Mr. Johnson: 알겠습니다.

Emily (Phlebotomist): 조금 따끔해요. 그러나 많이 아프지는 않아요. 제가 채혈하는 동안에 움직이지 마세요.

2분 후

Emily (Phlebotomist): 다 끝났습니다. 주먹을 펴도 됩니다. 채혈한 부위에 솜을 대고 누르세요. 하지만 문지르시면 안 되요. 약 5 분 동안 팔을 굽히고 계세요.

Mr. Johnson: 알겠습니다.

Emily (Phlebotomist): 혈액검사 결과는 약 40분 가량 걸립니다. 결과가 나오면 의사선생님과 함께 상의 하실 것입니다. 그 동안 대기실에서 기다려 주세요.

Mr. Johnson: 알겠습니다. 감사합니다.

4. Finger Prick /Finger Prick Blood Test
손가락 천자 혈액검사

손가락 천자 혈액검사

유아 또는 아동은, 란싯이라 불리는 날카로운 도구로 채혈을 합니다. 모세관으로 혈액을 수집합니다.

나의 혈액검사 이야기

제니의 손가락 천자 혈액검사

Patient's parent: 오늘이 딸아이의 혈액검사 예약을 한날입니다.

Nurse: 알겠습니다. 이름과 생년월일은 무엇입니까?

Patient's parent: 제니 스미스이고 07/09/2002입니다.

Nurse: 알겠습니다. 안녕, 제니! 앉아요.

Jenny: 네.

Nurse: 손가락에서 아주 작은 양의 혈액을 채취할 거예요. 먼저, 손가락 끝을 알코올로 소독하겠습니다.

Jenny: 어떤 손가락이요?

Nurse: 세 번째 또는 네 번째 손가락에서 혈액검사를 하고 싶은데요.

Jenny: 새끼 손가락은 어떨까요?

Nurse: 새끼 손가락은 검사에 적합하지 않아요. 왜냐하면 손가락 뼈가 다치는 것을 방지할 조직이 충분하지 않아서요.

Jenny: 와, 몰랐어요. 그러면 3번째 손가락에 할래요.

Nurse: 좋아요. 이것은 란싯이라고 해요. 란싯을 사용해서 손가락 끝에서 혈액을 채취할게요.

Jenny: 아파요?

Nurse: 조금 따끔해요. 벌침처럼. 엄마보고 안아 달라고 할까요?

Jenny: 네.

Nurse: 들어오셔서 아이를 안아주세요.

Jenny's mom: 알겠습니다.

Nurse: 제니. 세 번째 손가락을 아래로 향하게 잡고 손가락 끝에 콕 할게요. 준비됐나요?

Jenny: 예.

Nurse: 다 됐어요. 찌르는 부분은 끝났어요. 혈액을 수집하기 위해 모세관을 손가락 끝에 댈게요.

Jenny: 별로 안 아팠어요.

Nurse: 내 말 맞죠. 튜브가 다 채워졌어요. 검사가 다 끝났습니다. 그리고 아주 귀여운 반창고를 손가락에 붙여줄게요. 반창고는 오늘 이따가 떼거나 아니면 내일 떼어요.

Jenny: 네.

Nurse: 내원해서 고마워요. 잘 가요.

5. Oral Glucose Tolerance Test
경구당부하검사

경구당부하검사

당부하검사는 당뇨병을 진단하기 위한 방법 중 하나입니다.

가장 일반적인 당부하검사 중 하나가 경구당부하검사입니다. 경구당부하검사는 임신 24-28 주 사이에 임신성 당뇨검사에 사용됩니다. 검사 받기 전날 자정 이후부터 음식 또는 음료의 섭취를 금합니다. 그리고 검사 받는 중에도 음식을 섭취할 수 없습니다. 일정 양의 포도당이 함유된 시약을 마시게 됩니다. 채혈은 이 시약을 마시기 전에 시작되고 시약을 마신 후 30-60 분 간격으로 채혈이 시행됩니다. 검사는 약 3 시간 가량 소요됩니다.

나의 혈액검사 이야기

임신성 당뇨검사

산부인과에서

Doctor: 몇 가지 검사를 하겠습니다. 먼저, 경구당부하검사를 하겠습니다.

Patient: 알겠습니다.

Doctor: 이 검사를 받기 위해서는, 검사 전에 금식이 필요합니다.

Patient: 음, 얼마 동안 금식을 해야 하나요?

Doctor: 첫 번째 채혈을 하기 12시간 전부터 금식을 하셔야 합니다. 검사는 아침 이른 시간으로 예약이 될 것입니다. 이른 아침에 경구당부하검사를 받게 되면, 검사를 위한 채혈이 시행될 때까지 두 끼를 거르지 않으셔도 됩니다.

Patient: 배려해 주셔서 감사합니다.

다음날 아침

혈액검사 접수처에서

Receptionist: 혈액검사용지를 볼 수 있을까요?

Patient: 네. 여기 있습니다.

Receptionist: 경구당부하검사를 하기로 예약되셨군요, 그렇지요?

Patient: 예. 공복에 하는 검사라고 들었습니다.

Receptionist: 맞습니다. 언제 마지막으로 식사를 하셨습니까?

Patient: 어제 저녁 7:00 입니다.

Receptionist: 잘 하셨습니다. 채혈실로 가셔서 첫 번째 채혈을 하십시오.

Patient: 알겠습니다. 채혈실이 어디입니까?

Receptionist: 같은 층 복도 중간에 있습니다. 대기실 바로 옆에 있습니다.

Patient: 알겠습니다. 감사합니다.

채혈실에서

Phlebotomist: 성함과 생년월일을 말씀해주시겠습니까?

Patient: 서니 앤더슨이고 72년 2월 25일생입니다.

Phlebotomist: 알겠습니다. 앉으시고 이 용지에 서명하세요.

Patient: 바로 여기요?

Phlebotomist: 예. 용지 하단에요.

Patient: 다 됐습니다. 여기 있습니다.

Phlebotomist: 감사합니다. 몇 가지 검사를 하기 위해 채혈을 하겠습니다.

Patient: 알겠습니다.

Phlebotomist: 여기에 팔을 올려놓으세요. 토니켓을 팔뚝에 감고 채혈할 부위를 알코올 솜으로 소독하겠습니다. 조금 조이는 듯한 느낌이 들 것입니다.

Patient: 알겠습니다.

Phlebotomist: 주먹을 꽉 쥐세요.

Patient: 핏줄(정맥)을 잘 찾길 바래요.

Phlebotomist: 핏줄(정맥)이 잘 보여요. 걱정하지 않으셔도 되요..

2 분 후

Phlebotomist: 이제 다 끝났습니다. 이제 주먹을 펴도 됩니다.

Patient: 네.

Phlebotomist: 잠시 동안 누르고 계세요. 채혈한 부위를 문지르지 마세요.

Patient: 알겠습니다.

Phlebotomist: 만일 채혈한 부위에서 피가 멈추지 않는다면, 즉시 알려주세요.

Patient: 그렇게 하겠습니다.

Lab assistant: 이제 다음 검사를 위해 주황색의 설탕물처럼 단 포도당 시약을 드리겠습니다. 다 마셔야 합니다.

Patient: 혹시 포도당 시약을 마시면 속이 이상해지거나 그렇습니까?

Lab assistant: 맛은 좋지는 않지만, 속을 이상하게 하지는 않습니다. 걱정 마세요. 또한 경구당부하검사용지도 드리겠습니다. 포도당 시약을 다 마신 후 그 시간을 경구당부하검사용지에 기록하세요.

Patient: 알겠습니다. 포도당 시약을 마시겠습니다. 2시입니다. 이곳에 시간을 기록하겠습니다.

Lab assistant: 잘 하셨습니다. 이곳으로 2:30, 3:00, 그리고 4:00에 다시 와서 채혈을 하세요. 제가 시간을 적어드리겠습니다. 매번 채혈하기 5분전에는 도착해야 합니다.

Patient: 알겠습니다.

Lab assistant: 한가지 더 말씀 드리겠습니다. 이 검사가 다 끝날 때까지 물을 마시면 안 됩니다.

6. Lab Results
검사결과

검사결과상담

이상소견을 보이는 검사결과

Patient: 안녕하세요. 마크 앤더슨 입니다. 검사결과를 알기 위해 Dr. Kim 과 예약을 했습니다.

Doctor's office Assistant: 알겠습니다. 먼저 확인하겠습니다.

Mr. Anderson: 네.

Doctor's office Assistant: 앤더슨 선생님. 앉아계시면 담당 간호사선생님이 호명 할 것입니다.

Nurse: 앤더슨 선생님. 들어오세요

Mr. Anderson: 감사합니다.

Dr. Kim: 안녕하세요, 앤더슨 선생님. 병원에 오시는데 별 문제는 없었나요?

Mr. Anderson: 괜찮았습니다.

Dr. Kim: 다행이군요. 그나저나 몸은 좀 어떠신가요? 여전히 오심(메스꺼움)이 있나요?

Mr. Anderson: 없습니다. 처방 받은 약을 복용한 후로 위에 불편함이 없어졌어요.

Dr. Kim: 다행이군요. 음. 선생님의 검사 결과를 받았습니다. 그런데 추가 검사를 하려고 합니다.

Mr. Anderson: 결과가 안 좋다는 것인가요?

Dr. Kim: 아닙니다. 종종 검사결과가 명확하지 않아서 더 정확한 결과를 얻기 위해 몇 가지 추가검사가 필요합니다.

Mr. Anderson: 검사결과에 대해 지금 말씀해 주시겠습니까?

Dr. Kim: 확실하다면 말씀을 드리겠지만, 재검이 필요합니다.

Mr. Anderson: 결과가 안 좋은 게 확실하군요!

Dr. Kim: 며칠 후면 알게 될 것입니다. 걱정 마세요. 단지 재검하는 것입니다.

Mr. Anderson: 저도 그랬으면 합니다.

검사결과상담

정상인 검사결과

Patient: 써니 앤더슨 입니다. 혈액검사결과를 알기 위해 예약을 했습니다.

Doctor's office Assistant: 알겠습니다. 잠시만 기다려 주시겠습니까?

Ms. Anderson: 네.

Doctor's office Assistant: 앤더슨 선생님. 주치의가 기다리고 있습니다.

Ms. Anderson: 감사합니다.

Doctor: 안녕하세요, 앤더슨 선생님. 오늘은 어떻습니까?

Ms. Anderson: 많이 나아졌어요.

Doctor: 다행입니다. 오늘 아침에 검사결과를 받았습니다.

Ms. Anderson: 좋은 결과인가요 아니면 안 좋은 결과인가요?

Doctor: 좋은 결과입니다. 검사결과에서 비정상적인 소견은 없습니다. 혈액검사결과는 정상입니다.

Ms. Anderson: 아무런 문제가 없다는 뜻인가요?

Doctor: 맞습니다. 심각한 질환이 없습니다.

Ms. Anderson: 좋은 검사결과를 알려줘서 감사합니다.

Doctor: 별말씀을요.

7. Urinalysis

소변검사

어휘 퍼즐 정답

P	K	P	X	V	R	R	G	G	D	T	U	Y	D	W	V	J	U	I	V	B	O
G	V	P	I	B	H	B	X	V	C	O	R	U	Q	H	B	N	E	O	V	G	D
T	L	R	A	N	D	O	M		U	R	I	N	A	L	Y	S	I	S	X	K	Q
O	D	U	L	F	W	C	N	H	P	F	N	K	A	F	M	D	D	J	O	V	O
W	D	K	K	J	V	F	R	S	J	Q	E	F	W	P	N	F	S	H	X	K	C
U	A	E	B	J	C	P	X	S	S	T		S	O	Q	X	D	R	C	G	T	S
W	A	U	K	J	L	Y	C	C	T	G	S	L	E	I	U	P	E	S	D	Q	J
B	L	B	I	J	C	U	A	S	X	C	A	B	F	I	U	X	H	W	Q	K	O
T	V	A	R	G	V	L	P	K	R	S	M	L	X	R	L	H	K	K	Q	Y	U
K	P	N	P	M	Q	R	E	G	M	B	P	C	I	A	F	L	N	I	Q	D	M
N	S	N	R	Y	H	C	C	A	R	D	L	N	C	P	O	C	N	H	R	L	E
C	F	V	S	R	K	N	X	J	N	I	E	R	P	Y	I	X	Y	C	X	L	U
Q	I	Y	N	X	Y	O	E	Y	T			U	P	U	K	L	F	D	M	W	U
T	F	V	Y	U	B	Y	U	E	C	L	C	H	L	D	R	P	L	T	E	T	R
H	G	W	G	V	U	S	C	U	H	V	O	A	G	M	K	N	W	Q	O	K	E
R	K	D	U	R	W	R	L	D	N	F	N	V	T	N	P	G	O	F	L	T	B
S	G	S	I	G	R	T	H	R	C	X	T	W	Y	C	Y	B	J	E	U	J	U
Y	R	R	S	J	U	U	X	T	L	L	A	J	K	T	H	H	P	K	U	V	I
H	O	W	U	R	V	R	K	U	W	Y	I	T	F	J	N	W	X	L	Q	O	Y
G	Y	A	E	Y	D	N	H	C	L	Q	N	X	Y	W	O	J	W	L	Y	G	G
R	D	H	F	C	B	E	P	E	Y	M	E	L	E	Y	X	T	O	L	G	T	R
Q	K	N	K	J	A	I	C	J	E	N	R	V	Y	W	A	G	Q	Q	V	Q	N

void
urine sample
container
random urinalysis
clean catch
urine culture

독해구문

중간뇨 검체 채취방법이란?

중간뇨 검체 채취방법은 생식기부위에 있는 박테리아가 소변 샘플에 들어가는 것을 방지하기 위한 방법입니다. 이 방법은 일반 소변검사, 소변 배양 및 정확한 결과를 얻기 위해 오염되지 않은 소변이 요구되는 검사에 사용 가능합니다

소변검사관련 주요구문

검사에 관한 질문

Q1. 이것은 무슨 검사인가요?/이 검사는 어떤 검사인가요?

A1. 환자의 담당의사는 환자가 단백뇨가 나오는지 확인하려고 합니다.

A1-1. 담당의사는 환자가 요로감염이 있다고 생각합니다, 그래서 소변 검사를 하려고 합니다.

A1-2. 환자의 담당의사가 신장의 기능이 정상인지를 알기 위해 24시간 소변검사를 지시했습니다.

검사용기에 관한 질문

Q2. 왜 플라스틱 용기를 주는 거지요?/이 컵은 어디에 사용하는 것인가요?

A2. 환자의 담당의사가 소변검사를 원합니다. 그래서 이것은 소변 검체를 담을 컵입니다.

A2-1. 이 큰 병/주머니는 24시간 소변검체 용기입니다.

검체수집에 관한 질문

Q3. 어떻게 해야 하는 것인가요?/이 컵에 소변을 받아야 하나요?

A3. 평상시처럼 변기에 소변을 조금 본 후 멈추고 소변컵에 절반 가량 차도록 소변을 보세요.

A3-1. 이 검사를 위해 24시간 동안 소변을 모아야 합니다.

소변 검체 채집 후 검체용기에 관한 질문

Q4. 소변을 받은 다 받은 후에 소변컵을 어떻게 해야 하나요?/마치고 나면, 어떻게 해야 하나요?

A4. 소변컵의 마개를 꼭 막고 화장실에 있는 소변검체를 담는 트레이에 놓고 나오시면 됩니다.

A4-1. 화장실의 선반 위에 소변컵을 놓으면 검사원이 수거할 것입니다.

검사결과에 관한 질문

Q5. 검사결과를 알려면 얼마나 걸리나요?/검사결과를 즉시 알 수 있을까요?/언제 검사결과를 알 수 있을까요?

A5. 담당의사에게 검사결과가 전달되면, 결과를 환자와 상의할 것입니다.

A5-1. 며칠 후에 자세히 알게 될 것입니다.

A5-3. 검사 결과가 나왔습니다.

A5-4. 소변검사에서 이상소견이 발견되지 않았습니다.

8. Urine Dipstick Test
시험지 검사법

시험지 검사법

시험지 검사법이란 의사의 소견에 따라 전반적인 소변검사의 일부로 시행되기도 하지만, 그 자체로도 할 수 있는 검사입니다. 일단 소변 검체가 수집되면 간호사 또는 검사원이 특정한 시약이 묻어있는 시험지를 환자의 소변에 담급니다. 시험지에 붙어있는 시약 부분들이 백혈구, 단백질 또는 포도당의 유무에 따라 색깔이 변합니다.

나의 소변검사 이야기

시험지 검사(단백뇨 검사)

Patient: 소변검사를 받으러 왔습니다.

Lab Assistant: 알겠습니다. 먼저 몇 가지 확인하겠습니다. 성함과 생년월일을 알려주시겠습니까?

Patient: 린다 소토이며 1981년 6월12일 생입니다.

Lab Assistant: 환자의 담당의사는 환자가 단백뇨가 나오는지 확인하려고 합니다. 소변컵과 물티슈입니다.

Patient: 이 물티슈는 무엇에 사용하나요?.

Lab Assistant: 그것은 중간뇨 검체에 사용됩니다. 환자의 주치의가 단백뇨 검사를 지시했기 때문에 중간뇨 검체가 필요합니다.

Patient: 중간뇨를 어떻게 받아와야 하나요?

Lab Assistant: 그것에 관한 지시사항을 알려드리겠습니다. 우선 손을 씻으세요. 그리고 소변컵의 안쪽을 만지지 마세요.

Patient: 알겠습니다.

Lab Assistant: 소변 검체를 채집하기 전에 요도부위를 물티슈로 앞쪽에서 뒤로 한번에 닦고 물티슈를 버리세요. 두 번 반복하세요. 이해가 되나요?

Patient: 네.

Lab Assistant: 그런 다음 소변컵의 마개를 연 후에 소량의 소변을 소변컵이 아닌 변기에 보세요.

Patient: 처음 소변은 버리라는 뜻이지요, 그렇지요?

Lab Assistant: 맞습니다. 그런 다음에 소변컵에 1/3가량 소변을 보세요. 그리고 나머지 소변은 변기에 보세요. 다 끝나면 소변컵의 마개를 꼭 닫으세요. 이해가 되십니까?

Patient: 네. 다 끝난 후 소변컵은 어떻게 해야 하나요?

Lab Assistant: 화장실의 소변 검체를 담는 트레이에 넣고 나오면 됩니다.

Patient: 알겠습니다. 오늘 결과를 알 수 있나요?

Lab Assistance: 네.

9. Random Urinalysis
일반 소변검사

일반 소변 검체

일반 소변 검체는 하루 중 어느 때나 수집될 수 있습니다. 그리고 이런 유형의 소변 검체는 하루 중 특정 시간대에 소변에서 검출되는 다양한 성분을 검사하는데 사용됩니다. 종종, 이런 유형의 소변 검체는 특별한 조치가 요구되지 않습니다. 다른 유형의 소변 검체는 특별한 검사가 필요할 때 요구됩니다.

나의 소변검사 이야기

일반 소변검사

Nurse: 카운터로 검사용지를 가지고 오세요.

Patient: 여기 있습니다.

Nurse: 이름과 생년월일을 말씀해주시겠습니까?

Patient: 켄드라 버틀러이고 1977년4월27일입니다.

Nurse: 감사합니다. 검사용지에 따르면 담당의사선생님이 소변검사를 지시했습니다. 일반 소변 검체가 필요합니다.

Patient: 음. 일반 소변 검체는 어떻게 받아오지요?

Nurse: 일반 소변 검체를 채취하는 방법을 설명해 드리겠습니다. 먼저 변기에 소량의 소변을 보고, 잠시 소변을 멈춘 뒤, 소변컵의 약 절반 가량 채우세요. 이해가 됩니까?

Patient: 네.

Nurse: 여기 소변컵이 있습니다. 이름과 환자 인식번호가 소변컵에 적혀있습니다. 소변을 다 받은 후에 소변컵의 마개를 꼭 막고 화장실의 선반 위에 소변컵을 놓으세요. 검사원이 수거할 것 입니다.

Patient: 알겠습니다.

Nurse: 소변컵을 가지고 복도를 따라가 화장실로 가세요.
의료코디네이터가 그 곳으로 안내할 것입니다.

10. 24-hour Urinalysis
24시간 소변검사

24시간 소변 검체 채취

24시간 소변 검체 채취는 하루 동안 배출하는 모든 소변을 모을 필요가 있을 때 하는 검사입니다. 이것은 몸으로부터 신장이 걸러 내는 특정한 성분의 양을 측정할 필요가 있을 때 시행합니다. 일부 성분은 낮과 밤 동안에 다른 양이 걸러집니다. 24시간 소변 검체로 검사하려는 성분을 정확하게 측정할 수 있습니다. 24시간 동안 소변을 채취하려는 다른 이유는 소변 생산량이 너무 많거나 너무 적은지를 보기 위해서 입니다.

24시간 소변 검체 채취에 관한 지시사항

1. 24시간 소변 검체 채취 용기를 받으실 것입니다. 만일 필요하다면 냉장고 안에 또는 얼음 위에 보관할 필요가 있습니다.
2. 24시간 소변 검체를 채취할 때 항상 아침에 채취를 시작하세요.
3. 모으기 시작한 날의 첫 소변은 버리세요. 하지만 이 검사지의 아래 부분에 시작 시간으로 표기하세요.
4. 그 후 24시간 동안의 모든 소변을 모으세요. 정확한 결과를 얻기 위해서는 소변을 전부 모으는 것이 중요합니다. 만일 소변 채취를 거르셨다면, 의료진에게 자문을 구하세요. 가능하다면 검사 중에 6-8컵 정도의 충분한 물을 마시세요.
5. 마지막 소변 검체는 시작한 시간과 가능한 가까워야 하고 꼭 수집되어야 합니다.
6. 24시간 소변 검체 채취 용기를 냉장고 안 또는 얼음 위에 보관하는 것을 잊지 마세요.

7. 검체 채취 용기(들)을 ____________________로 가져오세요.

<u>아래의 정보들을 기입하세요:</u>

환자의 이름: ________________________________

채취시작 날짜: ___________시작 시간: ______오전/오후

채취종료 날짜: _________종료 시간: ________오전/오후

나의 소변검사 이야기

24시간 소변검사

Nurse: 의사선생님이 24시간 소변 검사를 지시했습니다. 24시간 소변 검체 채취에 관한 모든 지시사항을 말씀 드리겠습니다.

Patient: 알겠습니다.

Nurse: 우선 24시간 소변 검체 채취 용기, 소변컵과 24시간 소변 검체 채취 용지를 드리겠습니다. 집에 가지고 가세요. 환자의 이름과 환자인식번호를 용기에 적겠습니다.

Patient: 네.

Nurse: 다음 24시간 동안 배뇨하는 모든 소변을 검체 용기에 모으세요. 만일 소변용기에 첨가할 약품이 있다면 먼저 24시간 소변 검체 채취 용기에 첨가하세요.

Patient: 알겠습니다.

Nurse: 검사를 시작할 때, 아침에 소변을 보고 그 첫 소변은 버리세요. 그 후, 소변컵에 소변을 본 후에 큰 검체 용기에 부으세요.

Patient: 처음 소변은 버린다는 뜻이지요?

Nurse: 맞습니다. 하지만 그 시간은 용지에 기록하셔야 합니다.

Patient: 알겠습니다.

Nurse: 24시간이 경과한 후 배뇨한 소변을 한번 더 용기에 모으세요. 그리고 다음날 24시간 소변 검체 채취 용기와 24시간 소변 검체 채취 용지도 함께 가지고 검사실로 오세요.

Patient: 음, 마지막 부분이 이해가 안돼요. 24시간이 지난 후의 소변도 수집해야 하나요?

Nurse: 예, 첫 번째 지시사항을 기억하십니까? 처음 소변은 모으지 않고 버리되 시간은 기록해야 했지요. 이것이 24시간이 지난 후의 마지막 부분의 소변을 모아야 하는 이유입니다.

Patient: 이해가 됩니다.

Nurse: 만일 한 두 번 소변을 모으지 못 했다면, 검사실의 검사원에게 의뢰하여 추가적인 지시사항을 상담 받으세요.

Patient: 알겠습니다. 다음에 뵙겠습니다.

11. FAQ for the Lab Test:
검사에 관련된 자주하는 질문

자주하는 질문모음

검사절차에 관하여

Q1. 금식의 의미가 무엇인가요?

A1. 금식은 검사 받기 전 약 6-8시간 가량 물을 포함한 음식과 음료를 금한다는 것을 의미합니다. 환자는 금식기간에 약을 복용할 수 있습니다. 담당의사는 혈당검사 또는 지질검사를 위해 금식을 지시하기도 합니다. 하지만 모든 검사가 금식을 요하지는 않습니다.

Q2. 제가 익명으로 검사를 받을 수 있을까요?

A2. 예. 그 부분의 서비스가 저의 병원에서 가능합니다.

A2-1 현재 그런 서비스가 가능하지 않지만 곧 가능하게 되기를 바랍니다.

Q3. 검사실에 갈 때 무엇을 지참해야 하나요?

A3. 수납증을 가지고 오세요.

검사예약에 관하여

Q4. 검사를 취소할 수 있을까요?

A4. 예, 취소할 수 있습니다. 하지만 일단 검사가 시작 되면, 검사를 취소할 수 없으며 비용도 환불이 되지 않습니다.

Q5. 검사받기 위해선 예약을 해야 하나요?

A5. 예, 검사를 받기 위해선 예약을 해야 합니다. 저희 병원은 예약없이 내원하거나, 선착순으로 환자를 진료하지 않습니다.

Q6. 3시간이 소요되는 경구당부하검사의 예약절차는 어떻게 되나요?

A6. 환자가 내원 했을 때 3시간이 소요되는 경구당부하검사를 예약해 드립니다. 예약은 주중 오전 9시에 됩니다.

Q7. 만일 질문사항이 있으면 어떻게 해야 하나요?

A7. 만일 질문이 있으면 234-5678로 전화주세요. 전화 오는 순서대로 최선을 다해 답변해 드리겠습니다.

Q8. 검사용지는 얼마 동안 유효한가요?

A8. 검사용지를 처방받은 후로부터, 검사실에 내원해서 검사를 받을 일정한 기간이 있습니다. 이 기간이 만료되면, 검사를 받을 수 없습니다. 만일 그래도 검사를 원하신다면 담당의사로부터 검사 처방을 다시 받으셔야 합니다.

검사시설에 관하여

Q9. (혈액) 검사실은 어디에 있습니까?

A9. 병원의 주 검사실은 (일)층에 있습니다.

Q10. 어디에 주차를 해야 하나요?

A10. 검사일정이 있는 환자는 외래진료소 주차장에 주차할 수 있습니다. 검사실에서 가장 가까운 주차장은 (응급실) 옆에 위치해 있습니다.

Q11. 검사하러 어디로 가야 하나요?

A11. 의료코디네이터가 검사실로 안내할 것입니다. 그러나, 검사센터에 관해 질문이 있다면, 주저하지 마시고 전화주세요.

검사결과에 관하여

Q12. 언제 검사 결과를 알 수 있을까요?

A12. 검사에 따라 다릅니다. 긴급한 검사가 아닐 경우, 검사를 받은 후 (5) 근무일 안에 결과를 알 수 있습니다. 만일 긴급한 검사일 경우 한 시간 내에 병원에서 결과를 알 수가 있습니다.

Q13. 검사결과가 비공개인가요?

A13. 환자의 동의 없이 의료기록을 제 3 자와 공유하지 않습니다. 환자의 개인정보 보호 정책을 준수합니다.

Q14. 검사결과가 무엇을 의미하는지 어떻게 알지요?

A14. 대부분의 검사는 정상범위 수치가 있습니다. 만일 검사결과 수치가 정상범위가 아닐 경우, 담당의사가 검사결과에 대해 환자에게 설명해 드릴 것입니다.

Q15. 검사 결과의 신뢰도는 어느 정도 인가요?

A15. 우리 병원은 과학적으로 입증된 검사 방법을 사용하여 신뢰할 수 있는 검사를 제공합니다. 그러나 검체의 정확성에 영향을 미치는 몇 가지 문제들이 제기 됩니다. 예를 들면, 일부 검사는 금식을 요합니다, 그러나 만일 금식을 하지 않았다면 검사 결과는 정확하지 않게 됩니다. 다른 문제는 검체 자체를 어떻게 처리하느냐에 달려있습니다. 만일 검사결과가 정확하지 않다고 생각된다면, 재검사를 받을 것을 권유합니다.

Q16. 검사결과 사본을 받을 수 있나요?

A16. 예. 검사결과의 사본이 필요하다면, 우편 또는 팩스로 보내드릴 수 있습니다.

Q17. 만일 내 검사결과지를 잃어버렸다면, 사본을 받을 수 있을까요?

A17. 만일 검사결과지를 잃어버렸다면, 다시 결과지를 발급해서 보내드릴 수 있습니다.

검사비용에 관하여

Q18. 현찰 이외에 다른 것으로도 지불이 가능합니까?

A18. 신용카드도 받습니다.

Q19. 국제의료보험도 받습니까?

A19. 모든 국제 보험은 아니나 일부 국제보험을 받습니다. 또한, 만일 환자의 국제의료보험이 우리 병원과 계약이 되어있지 않거나 직접청구방법으로 체결되지 않았다면, 모든 비용을 본인이 부담하여 자비로 지불하셔야 합니다.

Q20. 제 보험청구서를 작성해 주실 수 있습니까?

A20. 해드릴 수 있습니다. 그러나 보험료를 받기 위해서는 본인이 보험회사에 청구서를 보내야 할 것입니다..

Chapter 8

X-ray Examination

방사선 검사

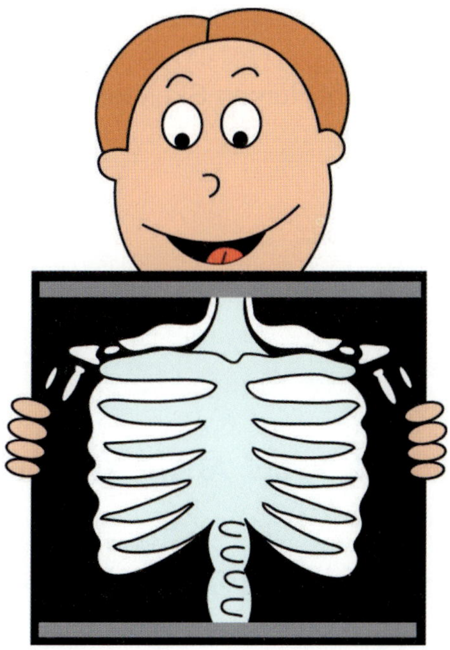

1. X-ray Examination
방사선 검사

- **Key words, 주요어휘**
  - QUIZ: 내 단어장 점검하기
  - Drill: Word Search Puzzle, 연습문제: 어휘퍼즐
- **The Human Skeleton, 인체골격구조**
  - The Main Bones of Human Skeleton, 주요 인체골격구조
  - Words, 어휘
  - Test Your Self, 자가진단
- **Reading material: Facts About X-ray Examination, 독해구문: 방사선 검사에 관하여**
  - Words, 어휘

· ***Code Breaker's Corner, 로리와 함께하는 미국 문화 엿보기***

■ Hospital Gown In America, 미국 병원의 환자복

· **Key Expressions for X-ray Examination, 방사선 검사관련 주요구문**

■ Words, 어휘

■ Drill, 연습문제

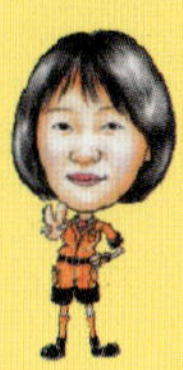

이 책의 녹음 파일은 www.ohgieun.com 에서 무료다운로드 하실 수 있습니다

Key Words

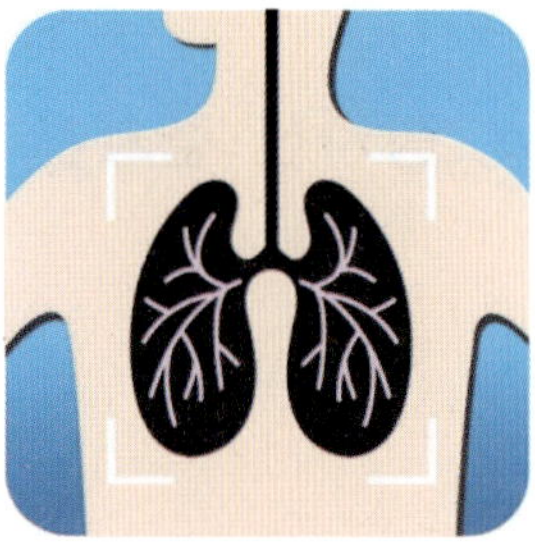

Chest X-ray: 흉부 방사선 (검사)

Abdominal X-ray: 복부 방사선 (검사)

Radiologist: 영상의학과 전문의

X-ray Table: 방사선 영상 촬영 테이블

X-ray lab/X-ray room: 방사선 검사실

Radiotechnologist (Radiographer): 방사선사

X-ray Appointment Slip: 방사선 검사 예약용지

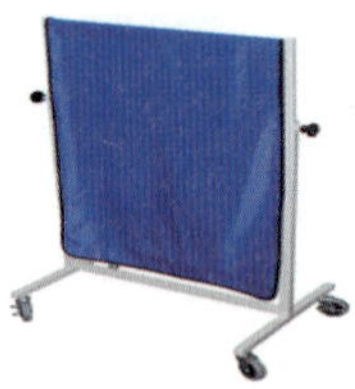

Lead shield: 방사선 차폐막

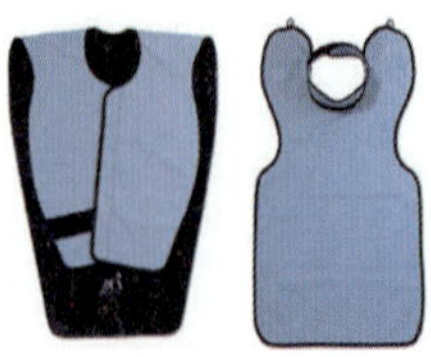

Lead apron: 차폐 앞치마

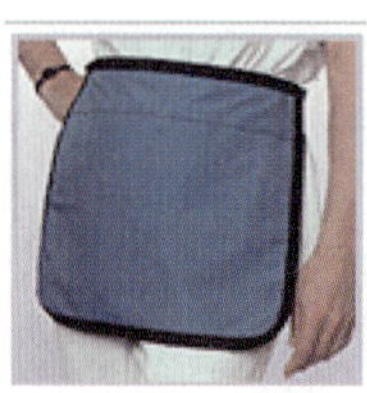

Half lead apron: 짧은 차폐 앞치마

QUIZ: 내 단어장 점검하기 !!

아래 단어를 읽고 알맞은 뜻을 적어보세요.

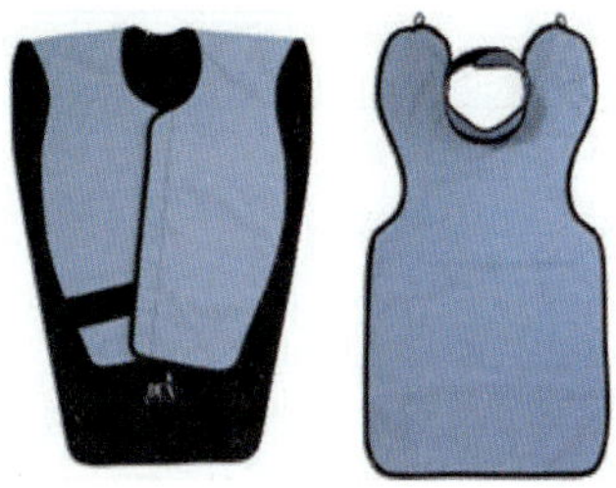

Chest X-ray: ....

Abdominal X-ray: ....

Radiologist: ....

X-ray Table: ....

X-ray lab/X-ray room: ....

Radiotechnologist (Radiographer): ....

X-ray Appointment Slip: ....

Lead apron: ....

Lead shield: ....

Half lead apron: ....

Drill: 아래의 단어를 ***Word Search Puzzle***에서 찾아보세요.

B	D	S	Q	R	Q	R	F	X	T	X	G	J	F	U	P	M
R	U	Y	G	Y	O	A	E	J	X	W	K	H	N	H	N	R
N	Q	G	D	I	U	D	X	F	G	E	K	Q	Y	F	U	D
E	P	B	S	E	K	I	W	C	S	J	L	N	M	Q	X	H
D	E	U	B	C	R	O	F	V	N	F	J	H	F	O		Q
L	L	I	T	I	H	T	P	W	P	R	V	Q	C	L	R	X
P	M	R	D	V	P	E	U	P	C	E	G	B	U	L	A	K
D	W	E	A	H	Y	C	S	T	S	G	A	Q	U	T	Y	B
X	A	B	R	D	I	H	P	T	P	Y	Q	W	I	X		C
A	B	D	O	M	I	N	A	L		X		R	A	Y	R	K
T	W	O	O	X	E	O	W	S	S	X	Q	O	F	H	O	H
W	H	I	E	Y	J	L	L	E	A	D		A	P	R	O	N
B	G	U	P	T	X	O	G	O	Q	S	N	R	G	E	M	I
V	L	X	E	Q	O	G	I	M	G	M	T	D	A	E	I	R
N	X	C	F	O	H	I	J	N	U	I	T	H	G	Y	B	F
A	L	O	E	A	R	S	H	J	F	L	S	R	Y	U	D	J
U	R	F	J	V	V	T	D	J	V	T	F	T	X	S	B	Q

영상의학과 전문의, 차폐 앞치마, 복부 방사선 (검사),
흉부 방사선 (검사), 방사선사, 방사선 검사실

The Human Skeleton

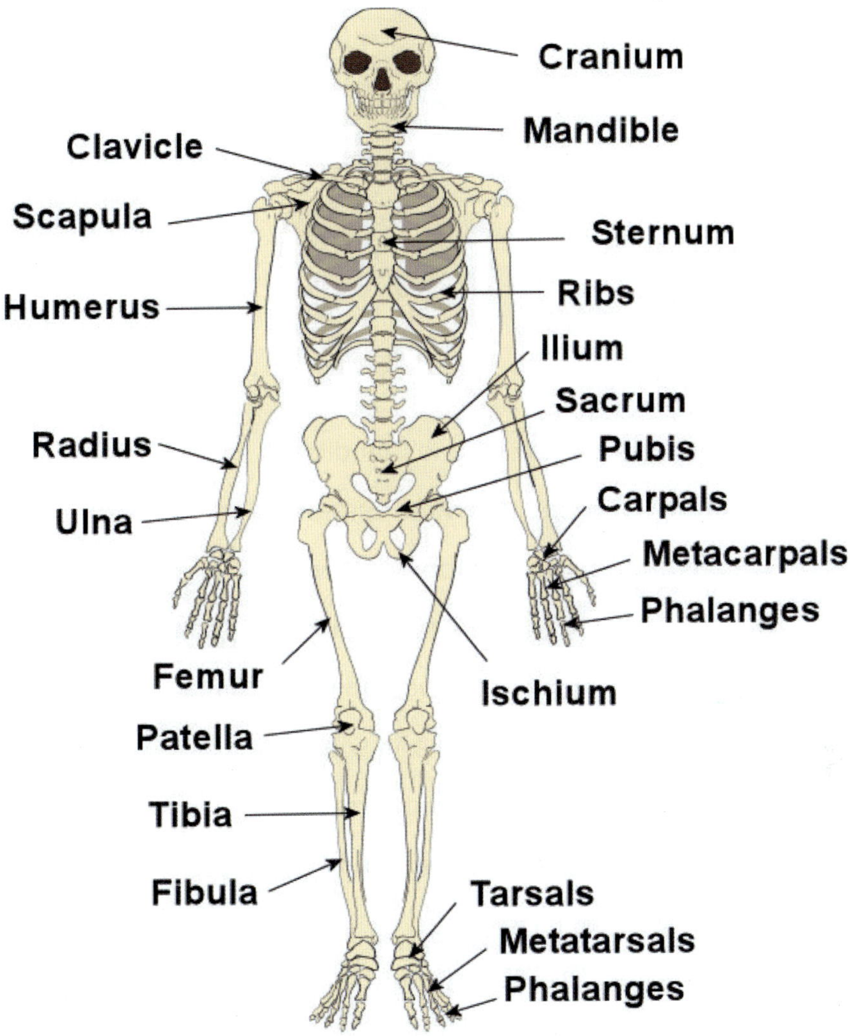

The Main Bones of Human Skeleton

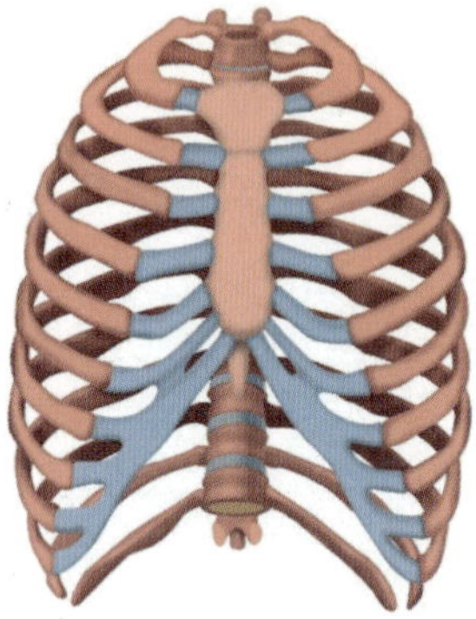

Skull-Cranium, Maxilla and Mandible

Vertebral Column - Cervical vertebrae, Thoracic vertebrae, Lumbar vertebrae, Sacrum (5 fused or stuck together bones) and Coccyx (the tiny bit at the bottom of the spine).

Shoulder girdle - clavicle and scapula

Arm - Humerus, Radius and Ulna

Hand - Carpals, Metacarpals and Phalanges

Chest - Sternum and Ribs

Pelvic girdle - Ilium, Pubis and Ischium

Leg - Femur, Tibia and Fibula

Ankle - Talus and Calcaneus

Foot - Tarsals, Metatarsals and Phalanges

Words

Skull: 머리뼈

Cranium: 두개골

Maxilla: 위턱뼈/상악골

Mandible: 아래턱뼈/하악골

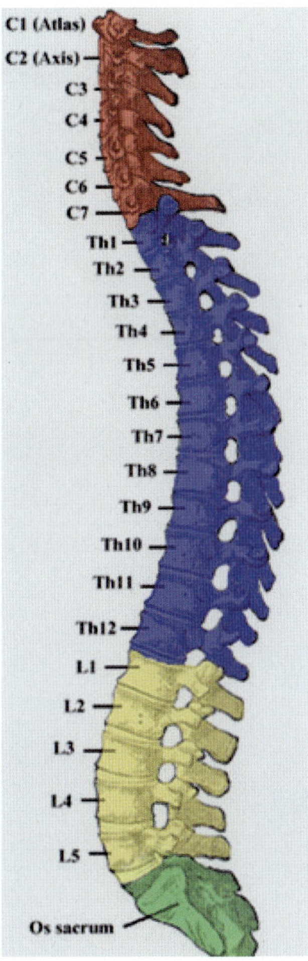

Vertebral Column: 척주

Cervical vertebrae: 목뼈/경추

Thoracic vertebrae: 등뼈/흉추

Lumbar vertebrae: 허리뼈/요추

Sacrum (5 fused or stuck together bones): 엉치뼈/천추 (5개의 융합된 뼈)

Coccyx (the tiny bit at the bottom of the Vertebral Column): 꼬리뼈/미추 (척주의 마지막부분에 위치한 작은 부분)

Shoulder girdle: 견갑대

Clavicle: 빗장뼈/쇄골

Scapula: 어깨뼈/견갑골

Humerus: 위 팔뼈/상완골

Chapter 8

Radius: 노뼈/요골

Ulna: 자뼈/척골

Carpals: 손목, 손목뼈/수근골

Metacarpals:손허리뼈/중수골

Phalanges: 손가락뼈/지절골

Sternum: 복장뼈/흉골

Ribs: 갈비뼈/늑골

Pelvic girdle: 골반대

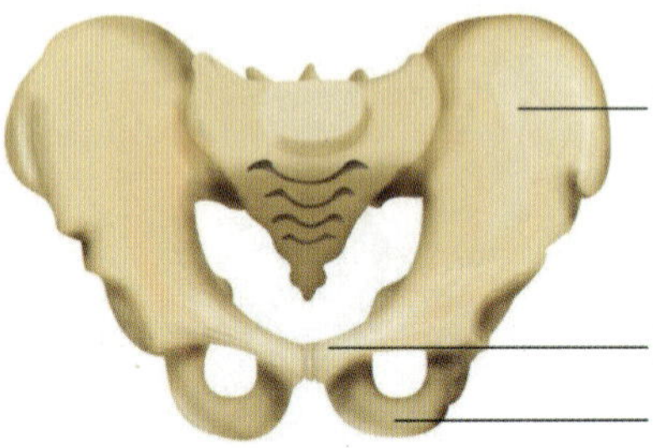

Ilium: 엉덩뼈/장골

Pubis: 두덩뼈/치골

Ischium: 궁둥뼈/좌골

Femur: 넓다리뼈/대퇴골

Patella: 무릎뼈/슬개골

Tibia: 정강뼈/경골

Fibula: 종아리뼈/비골

Talus: 목말뼈/거골

Calcaneus: 발꿈치뼈/종골

Tarsals: 발목뼈/발족근골

Metatarsals:발허리뼈/중족골

Phalanges: 발가락뼈/지골

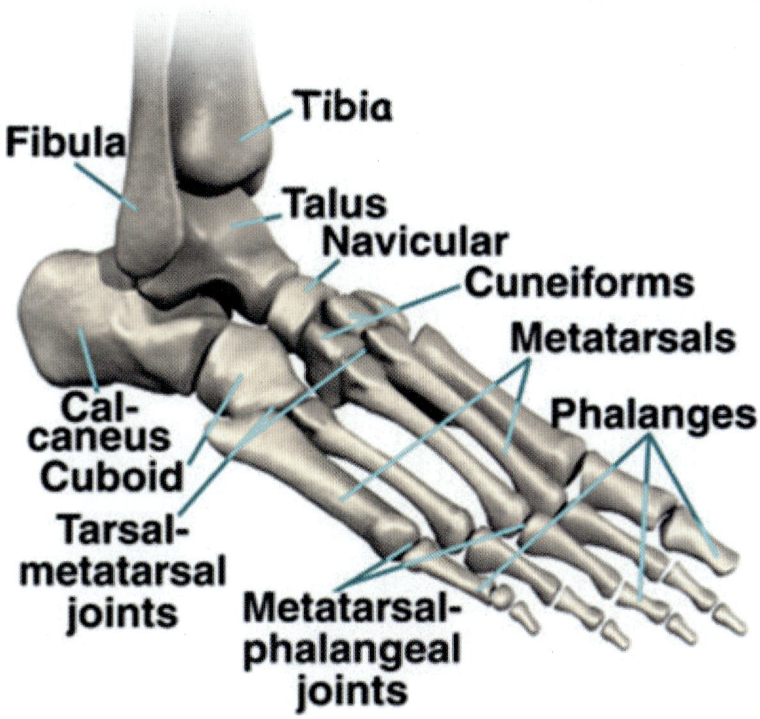

Test Yourself

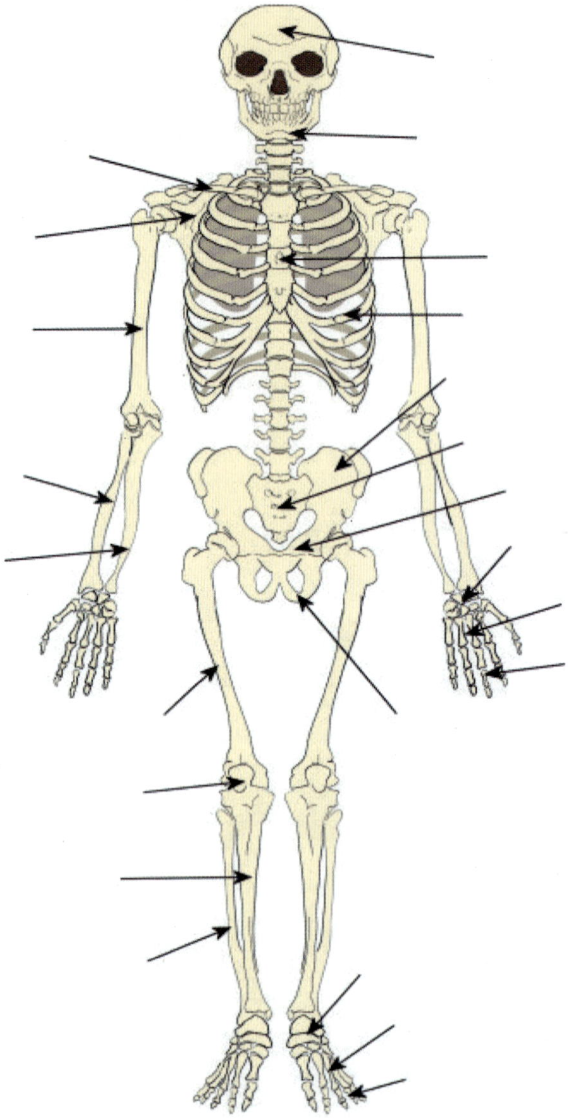

Reading Material

Facts About X-ray Examination

In the X-ray Department

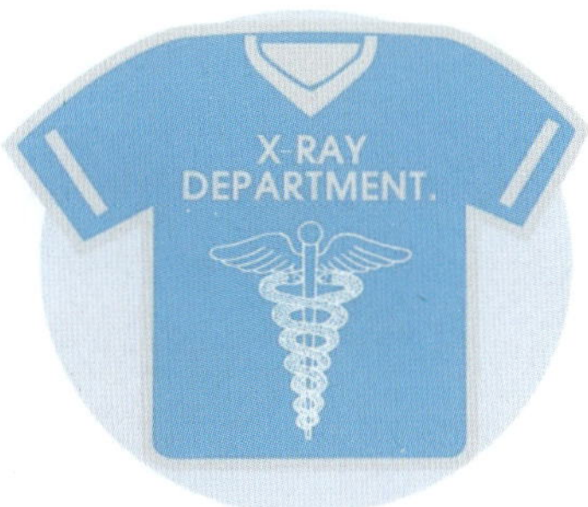

Welcome to the X-ray room. You may be having a hand, a foot, your chest, your back and/or any other part of your body X-rayed.

Patient Preparation

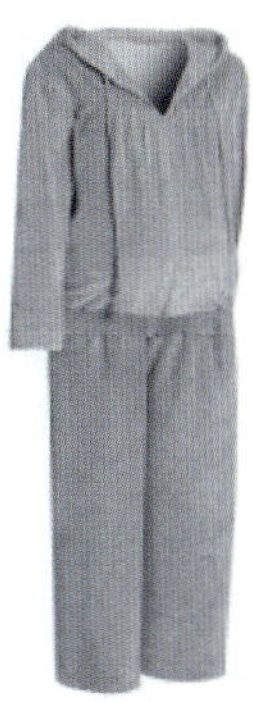

Outpatient: Wear a comfortable, 2-piece outfit on the day of your chest X-ray examination. Prior to performing your examination, healthcare provider will give you a hospital gown to wear.
This gown has no metal snap buttons on it because metal can interfere with the accuracy of the image.

Reading Material

Your Hairdo

If you have long hair and it is in a low pony tail, the elastic band or barrette may have to be removed as well.

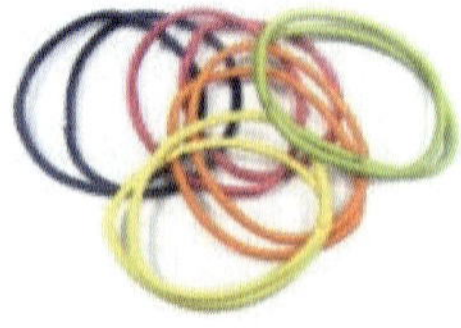

Elastic band

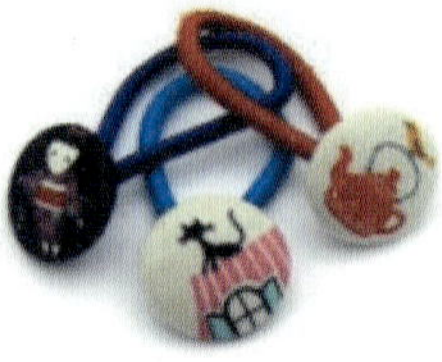

Hair bobble

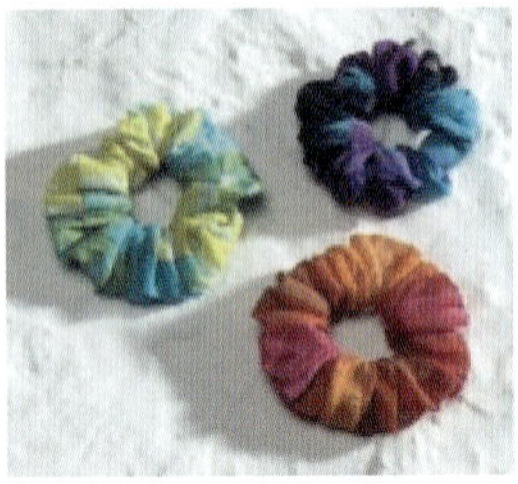

Hair scrunchy

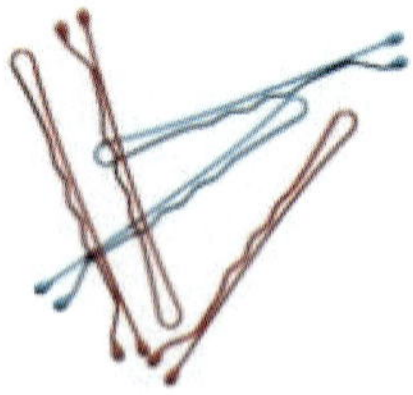

Bobby pin

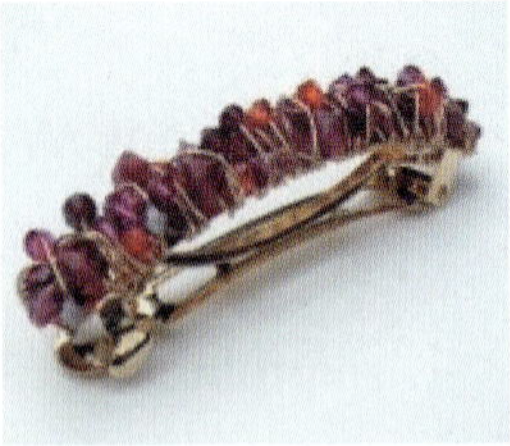

Barrette

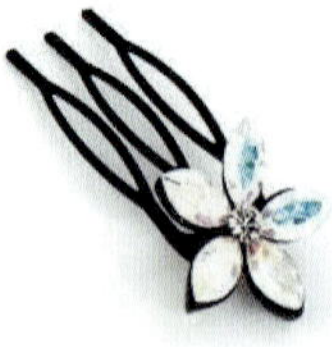

Hair comb

Reading Material

Personal Belongings

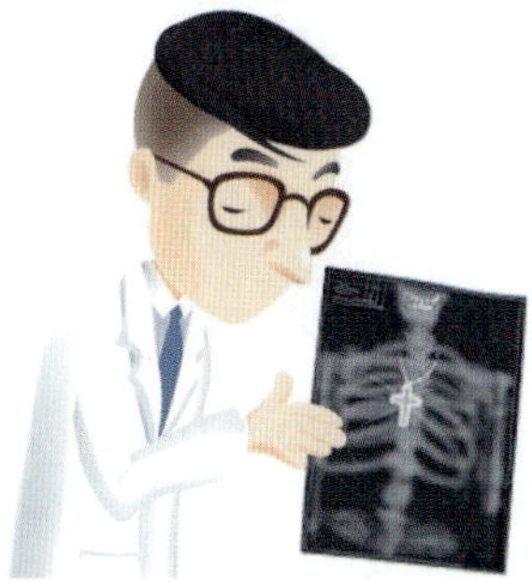

It is important that you remove everything from the waist up, including bras, undershirts, necklaces and other jewelry.

Pregnancy

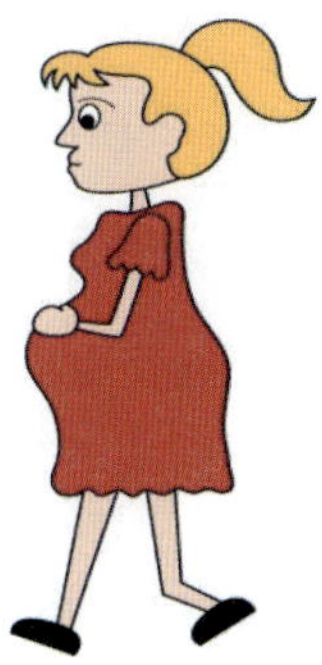

If you are a woman of childbearing age, it is important that you tell the radiographer whether you are pregnant. Pregnant women, if possible, should not have an X-ray test as there is a small risk that X-rays may cause an abnormality to the unborn child. This is why women are asked before having an X-ray if they are, or might be, pregnant.

Reading Material

During the Examination

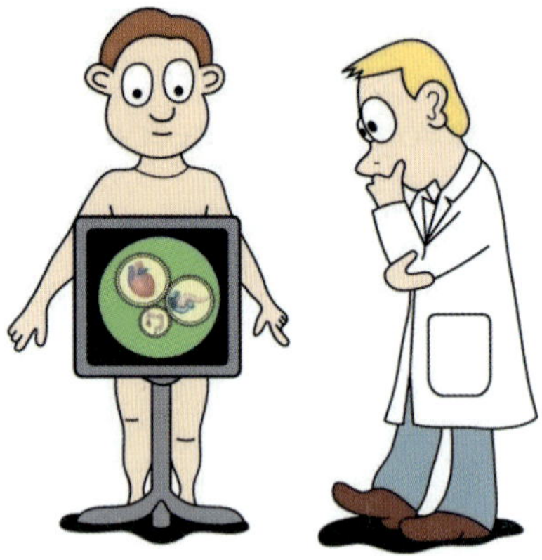

There is no discomfort during the examination. The films are taken while you are lying on your back, side, and while you are standing.

Post Examination

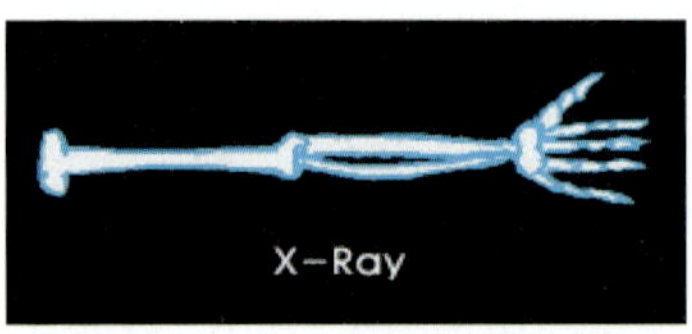

After your radiographs have been reviewed by a radiologist, your personal physician will receive a report and advise you of the results.

The radiation that you are exposed to during this examination, like the radiation produced during any other X-ray procedure, passes through you immediately.

Words

back: 등/허리 부위

outpatient: 외래환자

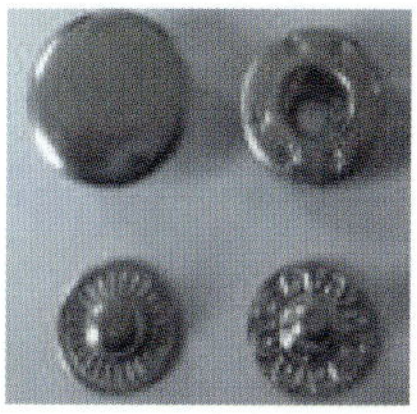

metal snap button: 금속성 똑딱(스냅) 단추

Hairdo: 머리스타일

low pony tail: 낮게 묶은 머리

high pony tail: 높게 묶은 머리

elastic band: 머리 고무줄

barrette: 머리핀

hair bobble: 머리 묶는 방울

hair scrunchy/hair scrunchie: 머리 묶는 것(일명, 곱창)

bobby pin: 실핀

hair comb: 머리 장식용 빗

childbearing age: 가임기 여성

lying on your back: 누워서

radiographs: 방사선 영상

pass through: 통과하다.

Code Breaker's Corner: 로리와 함께하는 미국 문화 엿보기

Hospital Gown in America

미국병원 환자복의 여밈은 앞이 아닌 뒤에 있지요......

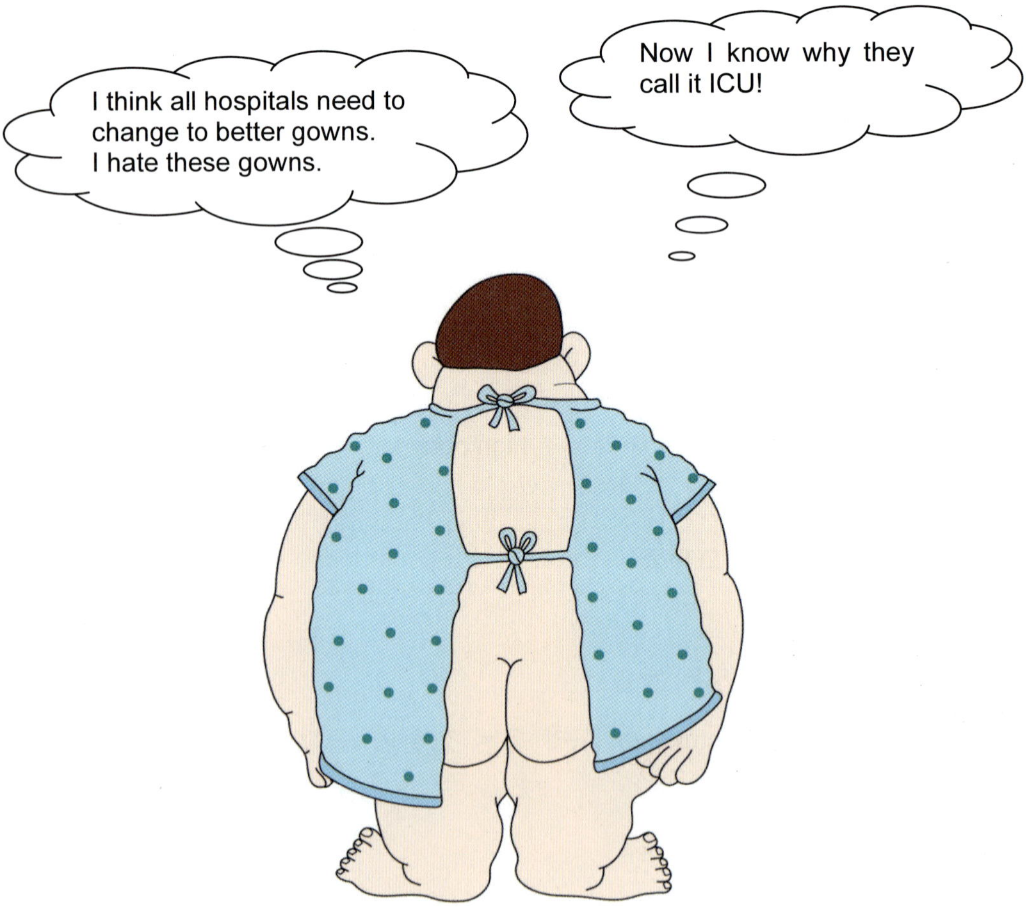
I think all hospitals need to
change to better gowns.
I hate these gowns.
Now I know why they
call it ICU!

ICU (Intensive Care Unit) vs ICU (I SEE YOU: 다 보이네!!!!)

Key Expressions for X-ray Examination

Step 1: ~부위에 방사선 촬영을 하겠습니다.

1. I will take an X-ray of your chest.
2. You will have an X-ray of your belly/abdomen.
3. I will take two pictures of your chest.

Step 2: 검사가운

1. Could you take your clothes off and put on the hospital gown please?
2. You need to take your clothes off and put this gown on, with the opening in the front please.

Step 3: 이쪽으로 오세요.

1. You will stand over here up against this board.
2. You need to come over here and face this board.

3. Please step on the foot sign and face the board right over here.

Step 4: 자세 교정

1. I will help position you.
2. I am going to put my hands on you to make a right position for your X-ray exam.
3. Would you please step backward a little?
4. Can you move a little to your left, please?
5. Please take a half step to your right.
6. Could you please lower your left shoulder a little?
7. Put your arms on your sides, please.
8. Please raise your arms to shoulder height.
9. Please turn your face this way.
10. Please take off your shoes and get on the table.
11. Lie on your back, please.
12. Please put your head on here and your feet down there.
13. We need to take a left side view, so please lie on your right side.

Step 5: 움직이지 마세요!

1. You need to hold very still while the pictures are taken.
2. Stay in that position, please.
3. Could you keep still like this for a second please?

Step 6: 숨을 참아주세요!

1. I am asking you to hold your breath for a few seconds to prevent a blurry picture.
2. Take a deep breath and hold it, please.
3. Now you need to take a really deep breath and hold it for a second please.

Step 7: 숨 쉬세요.

1. Now you can breathe.
2. You can let it out now.

Step 8: 검사가 다 끝났나요?

1. Is that it?
2. Will I be finished then?
3. Is that all there is to it?

Step 9: 옷 입으셔도 됩니다.

1. You will be able to put your clothes on as soon as I have checked the film.
2. That's it. You can get dressed when the film is developed.

Words

belly/abdomen: 복부

take your clothes off: 너의 옷을 벗다

opening: 옷의 여밈 부분

against this board: (흉부 방사선 촬영기) 보드 앞에

backward: 뒤로

a half step: 반 걸음

shoulder height: 어깨 높이

lie on your back: 등을 대고 눕다

blurry: 영상이 흔들린

Is that all there is to it?: 다 된 건가요?

Drill: Q1-Q34를 영작하세요.

정답은 전 페이지의 Key Expressions for X-ray Examination를 참고하세요.

1. 흉부 방사선 촬영을 할 것입니다.. ....

   ....

2. 복부 방사선 촬영을 할 것입니다. ....

   ....

3. 2장의 흉부 방사선 촬영을 할 것입니다. ....

   ....

4. Could you .... and put on the hospital gown please? 옷을 벗고 병원 환자복으로 갈아입으세요.

5. 옷을 벗고 환자복의 여밈이 앞으로 오게 입으세요. ....

   ....

6. You will stand over here up ....
   이 보드 앞으로 와서 서 주세요.

7. 이쪽으로 와서 보드를 향해 서 주세요. ....

8. 바로 여기에서 발바닥 그림을 밟고 이 보드를 보고 서 주세요.

9. 자세를 바로 하도록 도와드리겠습니다. ....

10. 방사선 촬영에 적절한 자세로 교정하기 위해 환자분의 신체에 손을 대겠습니다. ....

11. 뒤로 조금만 가 주시겠습니까? ....

12. 왼쪽 방향으로 조금만 가 주시겠어요? ....

13. 오른쪽 방향으로 반 걸음만 가세요. ....

14. 왼쪽 어깨를 조금만 내려 주시겠습니까? ....

15. 차렷 자세를 하세요. ....

16. 팔을 어깨 높이로 올리세요. ....

17. 얼굴을 이쪽 방향으로 돌리세요. ....

18. 신발을 벗고 방사선 촬영 테이블에 올라오세요. ....
....

19. 등을 대고 누우세요. ....

20. 머리는 이쪽에 다리는 저 아래쪽에 놓으세요. ....
....

21. 왼쪽 부위를 찍겠으니 오른쪽으로 돌아 누우세요. ....
....

22. You need to .... while the pictures are taken. 방사선 촬영을 하는 동안 움직이지 마세요.

23. 그 자세를 유지하세요. ....

24. 이 상태로 잠시만 움직이지 마세요. ....

25. I am asking you to ....
to prevent a blurry picture. 영상이 흔들리지 않게 몇 초 동안 숨을 참으세요.

26. 깊게 숨을 들이쉬고 참으세요. ....

27. 이제 숨을 깊게 들이쉬고 잠시 동안 숨을 참으세요. ....

28. 이제 숨을 쉬셔도 됩니다. ....

29. 숨을 내 쉬셔도 됩니다. ....

30. 다 끝났나요? ....

31. 검사가 다 끝난 거죠? ....

32. 다 된 건가요? ....

33. You will be able to ....
영상을 확인한 후 곧바로 옷을 입으실 수 있습니다.

34. 다 되었습니다. 영상이 나오면 곧 옷을 입을 수 있습니다. ......

2. Chest X-ray Examination
흉부 방사선 검사

- **Reading Material: Facts About Chest X-ray Examination, 독해구문: 흉부 방사선 검사에 관하여**
    - Words, 어휘
- **Story of My X-ray Examination, 나의 방사선 검사 이야기**
    - Dialogue: Chest X-ray Exam, 대화: 흉부 방사선 검사
    - Words, 어휘
    - Review, 복습

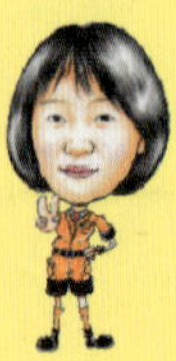

이 책의 녹음 파일은 www.ohgieun.com 에서 무료다운로드 하실 수 있습니다

Reading Material

Facts About Chest X-ray Examination

Chest X-ray

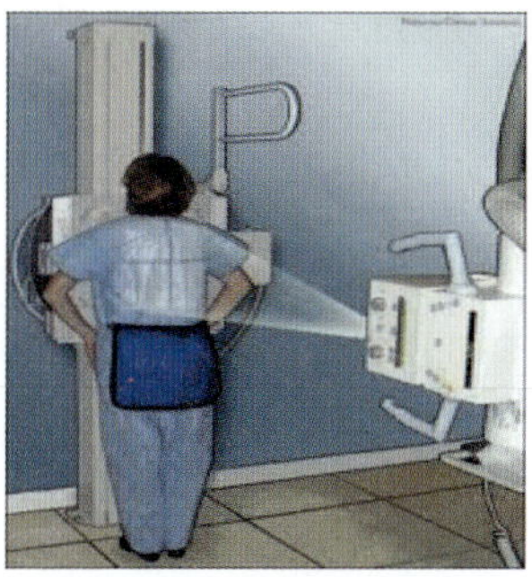

A chest X-ray is a photograph-like image of the heart and lungs that uses a small dose of radiation to create a picture. Two views are usually taken: the one is that the X-rays pass through the chest from the back (posterior-anterior view), and the other is that the X-rays pass through the chest from one side to the other (lateral view).

During the examination

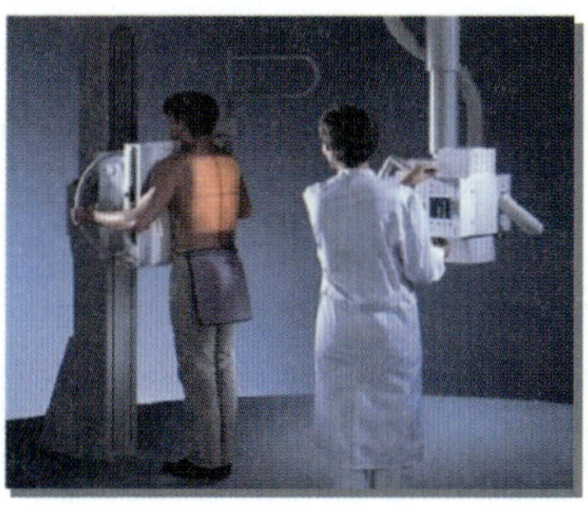

Inside the examination room, the radiographer will either hang a lead shield behind you at waist level or give you a half lead apron to tie around your waist. The thick rubber will protect your reproductive organs from direct X-rays.

Reading Material

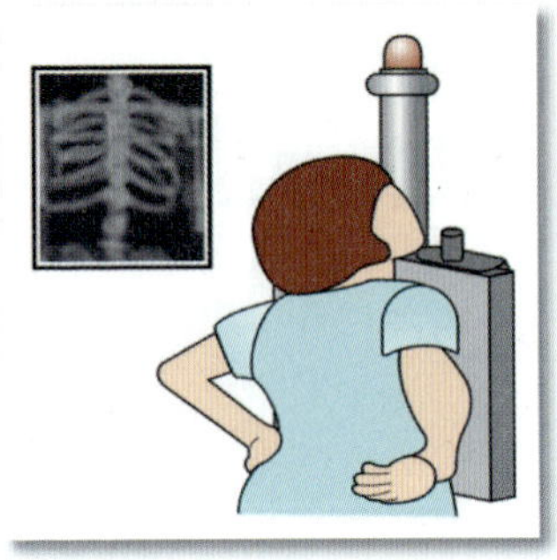

The radiographer will ask you to stand in front of an X-ray unit positioned at chest level. You will be asked to place your hands on your hips, roll your shoulders forward and lift your chin.

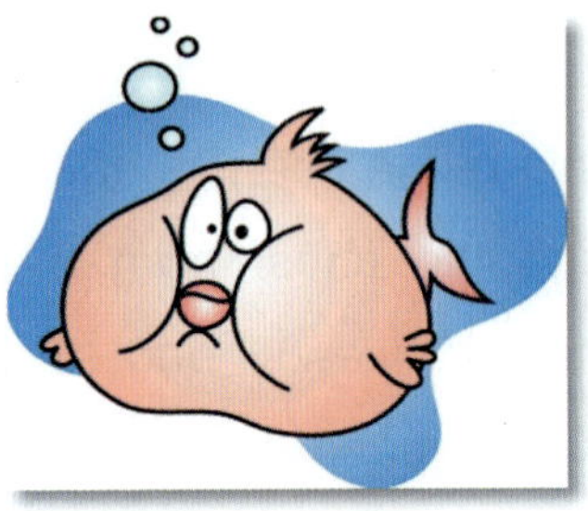

The radiographer then will ask you to take a deep breath, exhale, and then take another deep breath and hold it. It is important to hold your breath because any movement of your lungs will blur the X-ray image. The radiographer will make the X-ray exposure and let you know when you can exhale.

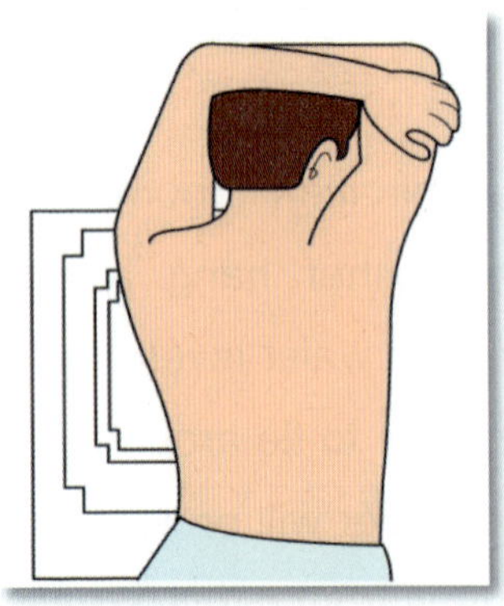

Radiographer will take the side view of your chest as well. Usually, you will be asked to turn to the side, and then raise your arms over your head and hold them in an upright position. Raise your chin again and hold your breath while the exposure is being made. The radiographer will let you know if more images are necessary.

Words

a small dose of radiation: 소량의 방사선

posterior-anterior view: PA view 가슴 앞쪽을 보드에 대고 뒤쪽에서 방사선 촬영을 하는 방법

lateral view: 측면에서 방사선 촬영을 하는 방법

lead shield: 방사선 차폐막

lead apron: 차폐 앞치마

reproductive organ: 생식 기관

chest level: 가슴높이

roll your shoulders forward: 어깨를 안쪽으로 구부려서

to take a deep breath: 숨을 깊게 들이 쉬세요

exhale: 숨을 내 쉬다

hold it: ~을 참다

blur: ~을 흐리게 하다

make the X-ray exposure: 방사선 촬영을 하다

side view of your chest: 흉부의 측면

turn to the side: 옆으로 돌다

upright position: ~을 위로 올린 자세

raise your chin: 턱을 올리다

Story of My X-ray Examination

Chest X-ray Exam

Receptionist: May I help you?

Patient: Yes. I need to take a chest X-ray exam.

Receptionist: Alright. Please go to the X-ray room, and your name will be called soon.

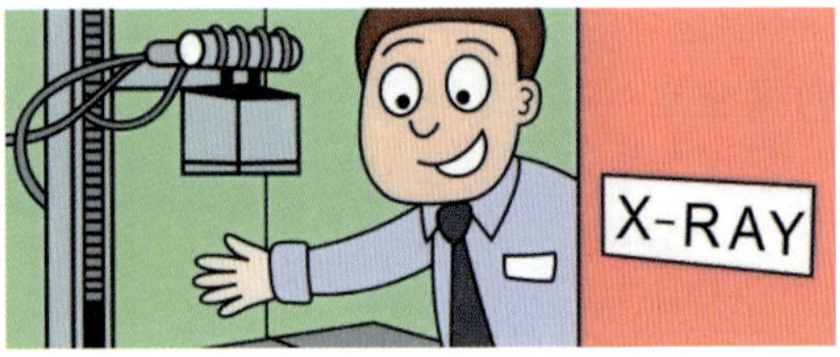

2 minutes later

Radiotechnologist: Hello. I am a radiotechnologist. Come in please.

Patient: Thank you.

Radiotechnologist: I need to verify a couple of things first. What is your date of birth?

Patient: 8/24/48.

Radiotechnologist: Can I see your Patient ID bracelet, please? I need to double check.
Patient: Sure. Here you are.

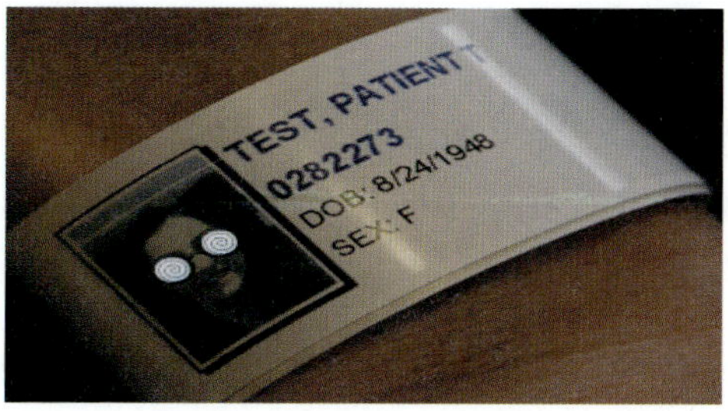

Radiotechnologist: Thank you. Let me check what your doctor has ordered for you today.
Patient: Okay.

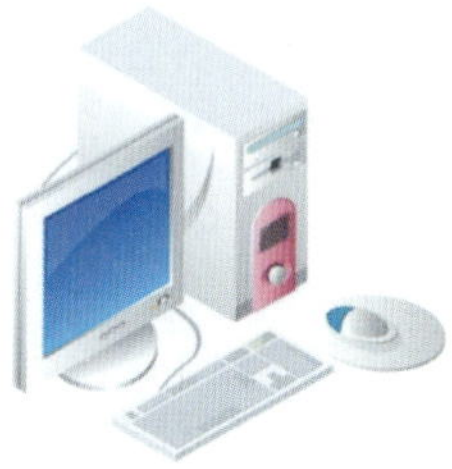

1 minute later

Radiotechnologist: Your doctor has ordered chest X-ray examination. First, you need to change into a hospital gown. Please come this way. This is the dressing room. Any question so far?
Patient: Yes. Do you think I can wear my underwire bra for the chest X-ray examination?

Radiotechnologist: Well, you need to take your bra off for the chest X-ray examination.
Patient: I see.

Radiotechnologist: Also, you need to put all jewelry and any metal objects in this container because metal or hard objects sometimes show on the X-rays and this might cause a wrong diagnosis.
Patient: Alright. Then I will put my barrette, necklace and cell phone in the container.

Radiotechnologist: After changing into the hospital gown, you can put your clothes and all the belongings including the container into the locker and lock it. Then hand me your locker key please.

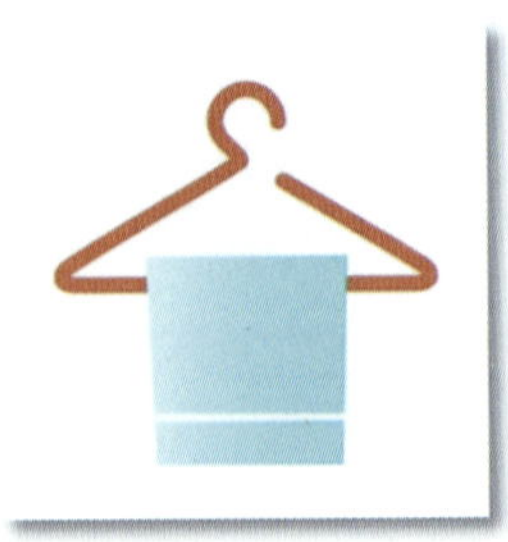

5 minutes later

Patient: Here's the key.
Radiotechnologist: Okay. Then, I am going to hang a half lead apron around your waist to protect your reproductive organs.

Patient: Oh, I see.

Radiotechnologist: Now, I'm going to take two pictures of your chest. Would you stand in front of the board please?

Patient: O.K.

Radiotechnologist: Please step on the "foot sign" in front of the board.

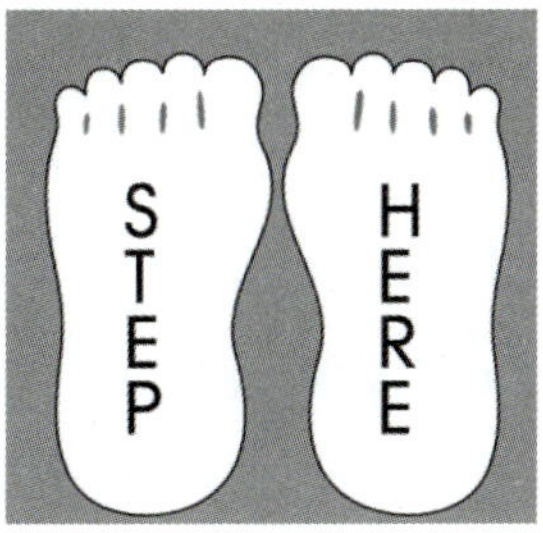

foot sign

Patient: Right here?

Radiotechnologist: That's right. Now I am going to give you some instructions. First, put your chin on here and place both of your hands on your lower back with palms up.

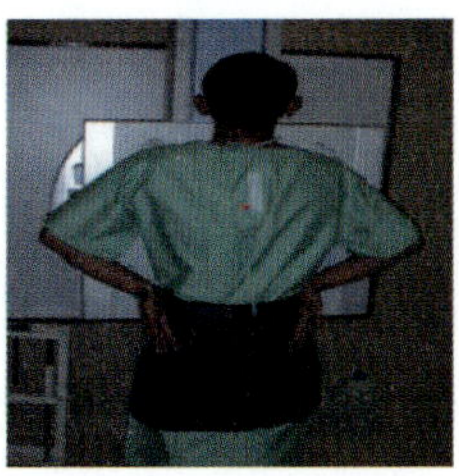

Patient: O.K. Like this?

Radiotechnologist: Great. Would you please push your shoulders forward? Please take a deep breath and hold it. Please keep still like this for a second.

Patient: O.K.

a couple of seconds later

Radiotechnologist: You can breathe now. Now, we need to take the second X-ray. The second X-ray is the side view of your chest. I am going to put my hands on you to help you into right position.
Patient: I see.

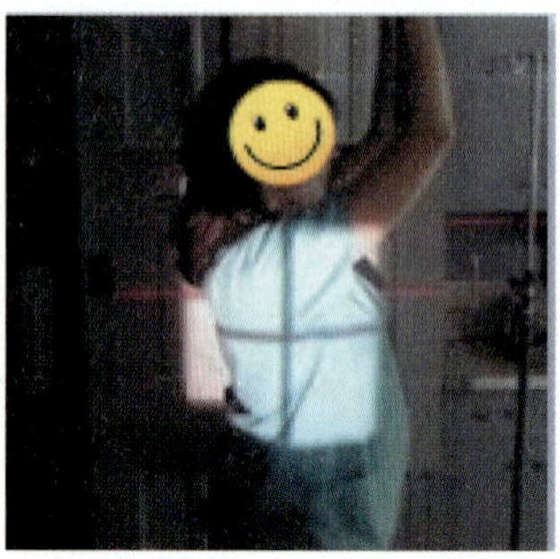

Radiotechnologist: Now you need to stand with your left side against the X-ray board with your arm raised above your head.
Patient: Alright.

Radiotechnologist: Stay in that position and take a deep breath and hold it please.

a couple of seconds later

Radiotechnologist: You can breathe now. Could you go out and wait a few minutes while I am checking your X-rays?
Patient: Okay.

Radiotechnologist: Unfortunately, we need to repeat your chest X-ray exam because they are blurry.
Patient: Oh, I see.

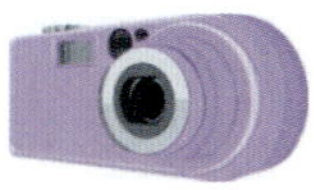

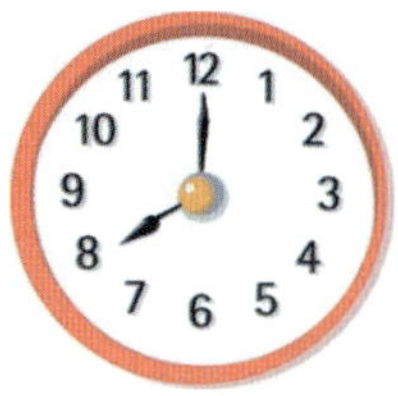

repeat the exam. 3 minutes later

Radiotechnologist: Your X-rays are fine. We are all through now. Here's your key and you can get dressed. After that you need to go back to your doctor's office, and your primary care physician will share the results with you.
Patient: I see. Thank you for everything.

Radiotechnologist: Thank you for coming in.

Words

dressing room: 탈의실

underwire bra: 언더와이어브라 (철사가 들어있는 브래지어)

container: 보관함

barrette: 머리핀

half lead apron: 짧은 차폐 앞치마

reproductive organs: 생식기관

forward: 앞으로

primary care physician: 주치의

Helpful Tips

Rib: 늑골

Lung tissue:

폐 조직

Spinal column: 척주

Heart: 심장

Chest X-ray

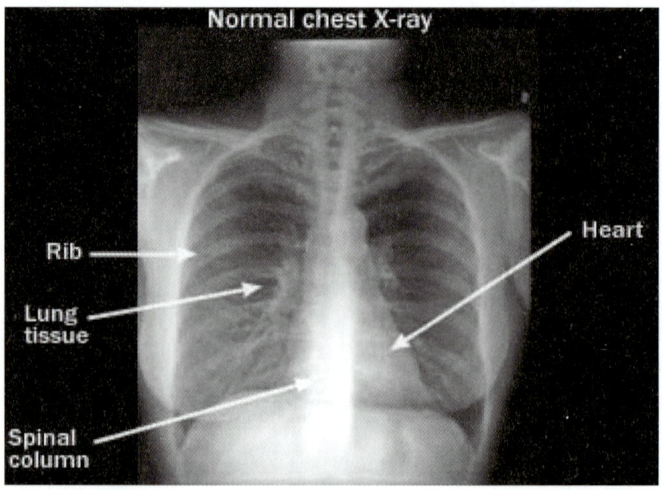

Review 각각의 구문을 영작하세요.
정답은 전 페이지의 Dialogue를 참고하세요.

Receptionist: May I help you?

Patient: 예. 흉부 방사선 검사를 받으러 왔습니다. ....

....

Receptionist: 알겠습니다. 방사선 검사실로 가세요. 그러면 환자분의 이름이 곧 호명될 것입니다. ....

....

2 minutes later

Radiotechnologist: 안녕하세요. 제가 방사선사입니다. 안으로 들어오세요. ....

....

Patient: Thank you.

Radiotechnologist: 우선 몇 가지 확인할 것이 있습니다. 생년월일을 말씀해 주시겠습니까? ....

....

Patient: 8/24/48.

Radiotechnologist: 환자 팔찌를 보여주시겠습니까? 재차 확인을 하려고 합니다.

Patient: Sure. Here you are.

Radiotechnologist: 감사합니다. 오늘 환자분의 주치의가 어떤 검사를 내렸는지 확인하겠습니다.

Patient: Okay.

1 minute later

Radiotechnologist: 환자분의 주치의는 흉부 방사선 검사를 지시하셨습니다.

우선, 병원가운으로 갈아입으세요. 저를 따라오세요. 이곳이 탈의실입니다. 질문사항이 있습니까?

Patient: Yes. Do you think I can wear my underwire bra for the chest X-ray examination?

Radiotechnologist: 음, 흉부 방사선 촬영을 위해 브래지어를 벗으셔야 됩니다.

Patient: I see.

Radiotechnologist: 또한, 모든 보석류 및 금속물질을 이 상자에 담으세요. ....

....

왜냐하면 금속 또는 단단한 물질들은 방사선 영상에 나올 수 있습니다. 이것은 오진을 야기시킬 수 있습니다. ....

....

Patient: Alright. Then I will put my barrette, necklace and cell phone in the container.

Radiotechnologist: 환자복으로 갈아입은 후에 옷과 보관함을 포함한 모든 소지품을 락커에 넣고 잠그세요. 그런 후 락커 열쇠를 제게 주세요. ....

....

5 minutes later

Patient: Here's the key.

Radiotechnologist: 예. 그러면 생식기관을 보호하기 위해 짧 차폐 앞치마를 허리에 두르시겠습니다. ....

....

Patient: Oh, I see.

Radiotechnologist: 이제, 흉부 방사선 영상 2장을 촬영하겠습니다.

보드 앞에 서 주시겠습니까? ....

....

Patient: O.K.

Radiotechnologist: 보드 앞의 "발바닥 그림"을 밟고 서주세요.

....

foot sign

Patient: Right here?

Radiotechnologist: 네. 지시사항을 알려드리겠습니다. ....

....

먼저, 턱을 이곳에 대시고 손바닥이 위를 향하게 양손을 허리에 놓으세요. ....

....

Patient: O.K. Like this?

Radiotechnologist: 아주 잘하셨습니다. 어깨를 앞쪽으로 당겨 주세요. ....

숨을 깊이 들이 쉬시고 참으세요. ....

잠시 동안 그 자세를 유지하세요. ....

Patient: O.K.

a couple of seconds later

Radiotechnologist: 숨을 쉬셔도 됩니다. 이제 2번째 영상을 촬영하겠습니다. ....

2번째 영상은 흉부의 측면에서 촬영하겠습니다. ....

....

촬영에 적합한 자세로 교정하기 위해 환자분의 신체에 손을 대겠습니다. ....

Patient: I see.

Radiotechnologist: 보드에 흉부의 왼쪽측면을 대고 서서 팔을 머리 위로 올려주세요. ....

....

Patient: Alright.

Radiotechnologist: 그 자세를 유지하고 숨을 깊이 들이 쉬시고 참으세요. ....

....

a couple of seconds later

Radiotechnologist: 숨을 쉬세요. 영상을 확인하는 동안 밖에 나가셔서 잠시 기다려 주시겠습니까? ....

....

Patient: Okay.

Radiotechnologist: 죄송하지만, 영상이 흔들렸기 때문에 촬영을 다시 해야 합니다. ....

....

Patient: Oh, I see.

repeat the exam. 3 minutes later

Radiotechnologist: 촬영이 잘 되었습니다. 검사가 다 끝났습니다. ....

여기 열쇠가 있습니다. 옷을 갈아입으세요. ....

....

그 후에 담당선생님의 진료실로 다시 가세요. 주치의가 검사결과를 알려줄 것입니다. ....

....

Patient: I see. Thank you for everything.

Radiotechnologist: Thank you for coming in.

3. Abdominal X-ray Examination
복부 방사선 검사

- **Reading Material: Facts About Abdominal X-ray Examination, 독해구문: 복부 방사선 검사에 관하여**
  - Words, 어휘

- **Story of My X-ray Examination, 나의 방사선 검사 이야기**
  - Dialogue: Abdominal X-ray Exam, 대화: 복부 방사선 검사
  - Words, 어휘
  - Review, 복습

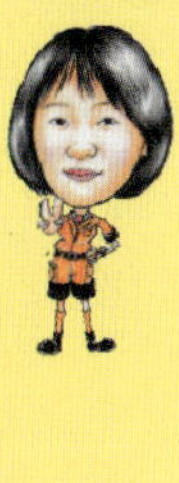

이 책의 녹음 파일은 www.ohgieun.com 에서 무료다운로드 하실 수 있습니다

Reading Material

Facts About Abdominal X-ray Examination

Abdominal X-ray

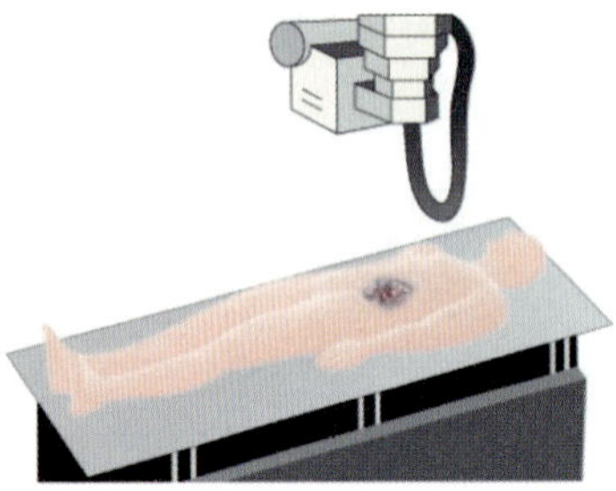

An abdominal X-ray is an imaging test to look at your organs and structures in the belly area, including the spleen, stomach, and intestines.

During the Examination

The test is performed in a hospital radiology department or in the health care provider's office by an X-ray technologist. You lie on your back on the X-ray table. The X-ray machine is positioned over your abdominal area. You hold your breath as the picture is taken so that the picture will not be blurry. You may be asked to change your position to the side or to stand up for additional pictures.

Reading Material

Precautionary Measures

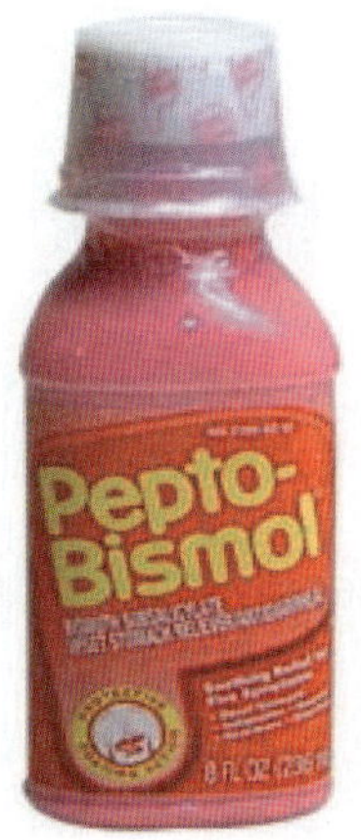

If you have taken any medications such as Pepto Bismol (which contains bismuth) within 4 days, you need to mention it to the health care provider. This type of medication may interfere with the test.

Words

belly area: 복부

spleen: 비장, 지라

lie on your back: 등을 대고 누우세요.

X-ray table: 방사선 영상 촬영 테이블

abdominal area: 복부 부위

blurry: 흐려지는

health care provider: 의료진

Story of My X-ray Examination

Abdominal X-ray Exam

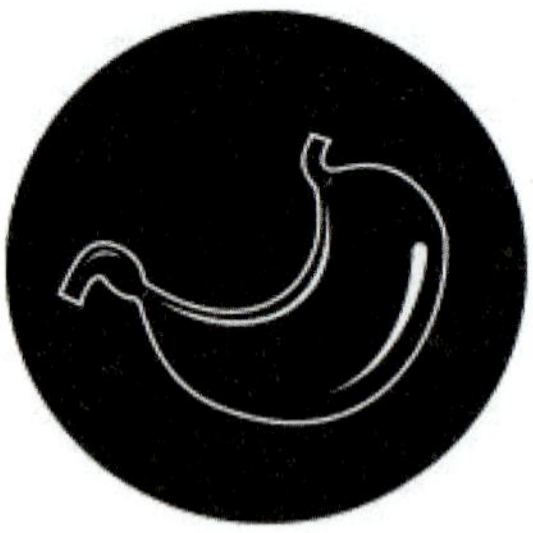

Patient: How long does the abdominal X-ray examination take?

Radiotechnologist: Actually, it takes no longer than 10 minutes. We need to take two pictures.

Patient: I see. By the way, should I change into a hospital gown?

Radiotechnologist: That's correct. The fitting room is right next to the X-ray lab. Here's your hospital gown. Please change into a hospital gown with the openings in the front.

Patient: O.K.

Radiotechnologist: Also, you need to put metal jewelry, cellular phone or belts in the locker because they may cover up structures in your abdomen. After putting all your belongings and clothes into the locker, lock it and hand me your locker key, please.

5 minutes later

Patient: Here you are.

Radiotechnologist: Alright. Would you please take off your shoes and get on the table and then lie on your back, please?

Patient: Right here?

Radiotechnologist: Yes. Please put your head up here and your feet down there. I am going to help position you.

Patient: O.K.

Radiotechnologist: Now, we are ready. If you move or breathe during the X-ray exam, the image may be distorted. So, please keep still from now on.

Patient: I see.

Radiotechnologist: Please hold your breath.

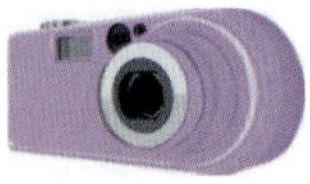

a couple of seconds later

Radiotechnologist: You can breathe now. We need the second X-ray. We need to take a left side view, so please, lie on your right side with your arm above your head.

Patient: Like this?

Radiotechnologist: Very good. Could you keep still like this for a second and hold your breath, please?

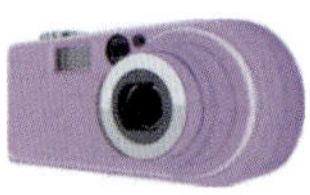

a couple of seconds later

Radiotechnologist: You can breathe now. We are all finished.

Patient: Well, it doesn't take much time.

Radiotechnologist: That's right. Thank you for your cooperation. Can you wait outside while I am checking your X-rays, please?

Patient: Sure.

Radiotechnologist: Your X-rays are good. You can get dressed. Here is your key.

Patient: Okay.

5 minutes later

Radiotechnologist: Now, you need to go back to your doctor's office. Then, your doctor will share the test results with you.

Patient: Alright. Thank you.

Words

fitting room: 탈의실

opening: 여밈, 트임

belts: 허리벨트

cover up~: ~을 가리다

keep still: 움직이지 않다

left side view: 왼쪽 측면

lie on your right side: 오른쪽으로 눕다

Helpful Tips

The Division of the Abdomen

Right upper quadrant: 우상부

Left upper quadrant: 좌상부

Right lower quadrant: 우하부

Left lower quadrant: 좌하부

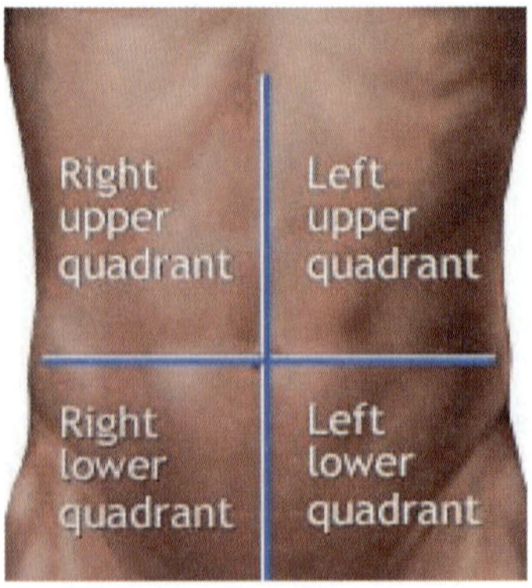

The Structure of the Abdomen

Liver: 간

Gall Bladder: 쓸개, 담낭

Pancreas: 췌장

Large Intestine: 대장

Appendix: 충수돌기

Spleen: 비장, 지라

Stomach: 위

Small Intestine: 소장

Bladder: 방광

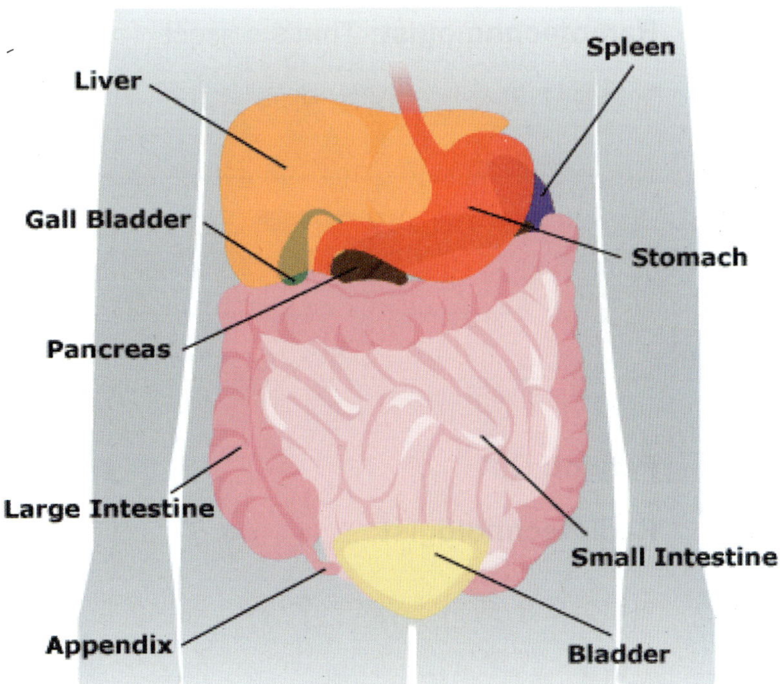

Review 각각의 구문을 영작하세요.
정답은 전 페이지의 Dialogue를 참고하세요.

Patient: 복부 방사선 검사는 얼마나 걸리나요? ....

....

Radiotechnologist: Actually, it takes no longer than 10 minutes. We need to take two pictures.

Patient: I see. By the way, should I change into a hospital gown?

Radiotechnologist: That's correct.

탈의실은 방사선 검사실 바로 옆방에 있습니다. ....

....

여기 환자복이요. 여밈이 앞쪽으로 향하게 병원가운으로 갈아입으세요. ....

....

Patient: O.K.

Radiotechnologist: 또한, 금속성 보석류, 휴대전화 및 허리벨트를 락커에 넣어 주세요. 왜냐하면 그것들은 복부의 장기를 가릴 수 있습니다. ....

....

개인 소지품과 옷을 락커에 넣은 후, 잠그고 그 열쇠를 제게 주세요. ....

....

5 minutes later

Patient: Here you are.

Radiotechnologist: 네. 신발을 벗고 방사선 촬영 테이블에 올라와 등을 대고 누우시겠습니까? ....

....

Patient: Right here?

Radiotechnologist: 예. 머리는 이쪽 위에 다리는 저쪽 아래에 놓으세요. ....

....

검사에 적합한 자세로 교정해 드리겠습니다. ....

....

Patient: O.K.

Radiotechnologist: 방사선 촬영을 할 준비가 되었습니다. ....

....

만일 검사 중에 움직이거나 숨을 쉬면 영상이 잘못될 수 있습니다. 이 상태로 잠시만 계세요. ....

....

Patient: I see.

Radiotechnologist: 숨 쉬지 마세요.

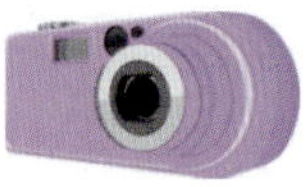

a couple of seconds later

Radiotechnologist: 숨쉬세요. 두 번째 방사선 촬영을 하겠습니다.

이제 왼쪽 부위를 촬영하겠으니 오른쪽으로 돌아 누우시고 팔을 귀에 붙이세요.

Patient: Like this?

Radiotechnologist: 맞습니다. 이 자세를 잠시 유지하시고 숨을 참으세요.

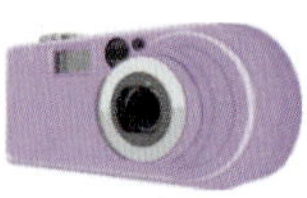

a couple of seconds later

Radiotechnologist: 숨쉬세요. 검사가 모두 끝났습니다.

Patient: Well, it doesn't take much time.

Radiotechnologist: 네. 협조해 주셔서 감사합니다. ....

....

영상이 제대로 나왔는지 확인하는 동안 잠시 밖에서 기다려 주시겠습니까? ....

....

Patient: Sure.

Radiotechnologist: 영상이 잘 나왔습니다. 옷을 갈아입으셔도 됩니다. 열쇠 여기 있습니다. ....

....

Patient: Okay.

5 minutes later

Radiotechnologist: 담당의사선생님의 진료실로 다시 가세요. ......

....

그러면 주치의가 환자분에게 검사 결과를 말씀해 줄 것입니다.

....

Patient: Alright. Thank you.

Pop Quiz: Identify the parts indicated by an arrow.

There are 9 questions in total.

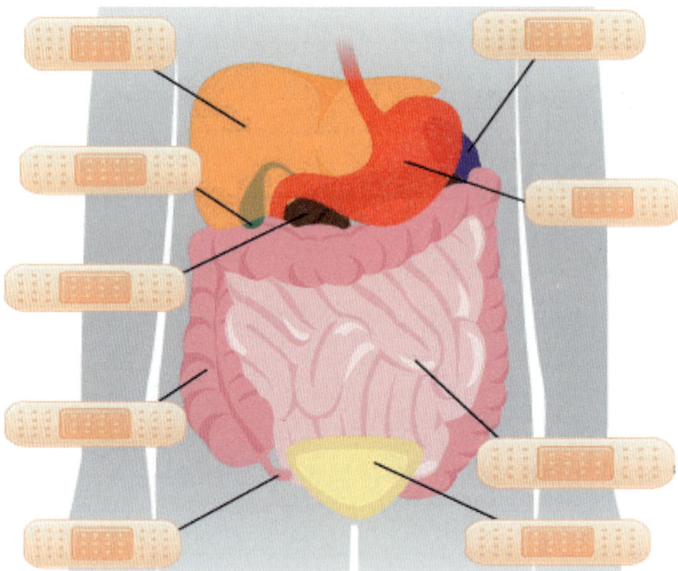

Word Review: 위의 단어들을 복습하는 공간입니다.
정답은 Key Words를 참고하세요.

뜻: In English

흉부 방사선 (검사): ____________________

복부 방사선 (검사): ____________________

영상의학과 전문의: ____________________

방사선 영상 촬영하는 테이블: ____________________

방사선 검사실: ____________________

방사선사: ____________________

방사선 검사 예약용지: ____________________

방사선 차폐막: ____________________

차폐 앞치마: ____________________

짧은 차폐 앞치마: ____________________

4. 해석 및 정답

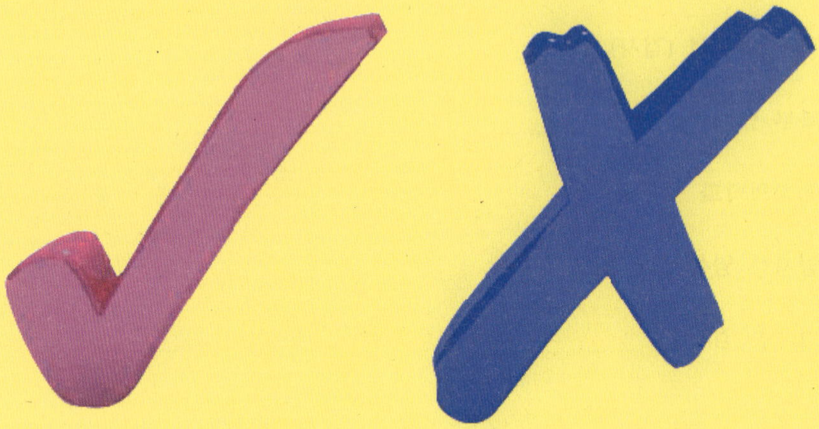

1. X-ray Examination

방사선 검사

어휘퍼즐 정답

B	D	S	Q	R	Q	R	F	X	T	X	G	J	F	U	P	M
R	U	Y	G	Y	O	A	E	J	X	W	K	H	N	H	N	R
N	Q	G	D	I	U	D	X	F	G	E	K	Q	Y	F	U	D
E	P	B	S	E	K	I	W	C	S	J	L	N	M	Q	X	H
D	E	U	B	C	R	O	F	V	N	F	J	H	F	O		Q
L	L	I	T	I	H	T	P	W	P	R	V	Q	C	L	R	X
P	M	R	D	V	P	E	U	P	C	E	G	B	U	L	A	K
D	W	E	A	H	Y	C	S	T	S	G	A	Q	U	T	Y	B
X	A	B	R	D	I	H	P	T	P	Y	Q	W	I	X		C
A	B	D	O	M	I	N	A	L		X		R	A	Y	R	K
T	W	O	O	X	E	O	W	S	S	X	Q	O	F	H	O	H
W	H	I	E	Y	J	L	L	E	A	D		A	P	R	O	N
B	G	U	P	T	X	O	G	O	Q	S	N	R	G	E	M	I
V	L	X	E	Q	O	G	I	M	G	M	T	D	A	E	I	R
N	X	C	F	O	H	I	J	N	U	I	T	H	G	Y	B	F
A	L	O	E	A	R	S	H	J	F	L	S	R	Y	U	D	J
U	R	F	J	V	V	T	D	J	V	T	F	T	X	S	B	Q

Radiologist	Lead apron	Abdominal X Ray
Chest X Ray	Radiotechnologist	X ray room

주요인체 골격구조

머리뼈- 두개골, 위턱뼈/상악골, 아래턱뼈/하악골

척주- 목뼈/경추, 등뼈/흉추, 허리뼈/요추, 엉치뼈/천추 (5개의 융합된 뼈) 및 꼬리뼈/미추 (척주의 마지막부분에 위치한 작은 부분)

견갑대- 빗장뼈/쇄골 및 어깨뼈/견갑골

팔- 위 팔뼈/상완골, 노뼈/요골 및 자뼈/척골

손- 손목, 손목뼈/수근골, 손허리뼈/중수골, 손가락뼈/지절골

흉부- 복장뼈/흉골 및 갈비뼈/늑골

골반대- 엉덩뼈/장골, 두덩뼈/치골 및 궁둥뼈/좌골

다리- 넓다리뼈/대퇴골, 정강뼈/경골, 종아리뼈/비골

발목- 목말뼈/거골, 발꿈치뼈/종골

발 - 발목뼈/발족근골, 발허리뼈/중족골, 발가락뼈/지골

독해구문

방사선 검사란

영상의학과

방사선 검사실에 오신 것을 환영합니다. 당신은 손, 발, 흉부, 등 및/또는 신체의 다른 부위에 방사선 촬영을 하게 될 것입니다.

환자 준비

외래환자: 흉부 방사선 검사 당일에 상의와 하의가 분리된 편안한 복장을 입고 오세요. 검사하기 전에, 의료진이 당신이 입을 병원 가운을 줄 것입니다. 금속물질이 촬영된 이미지의 정확도를 방해할 수가 있기에 가운에는 금속성 단추가 부착되어 있지 않습니다.

머리스타일

만일 머리가 길고 목 근처 부위서 묶었다면, 머리 고무줄이나 또는 머리핀 또한 제거해야 합니다.

개인 소지품

당신이 허리 윗부분에 착용한 브래지어, 속옷, 목걸이 및 다른 보석류를 모두 제거하는 것은 중요한 사항입니다.

임신

만일 당신이 가임기 여성이라면, 당신이 임신을 했을 가능성에 관하여 방사선사에게 말하는 것은 중요합니다. 방사선 검사가 태아에게 기형을 유발할 수 있으므로, 가능하다면 임산부는 방사선 검사를 하지 말아야 합니다. 이런 이유로 방사선 검사를 하기 전에 여성들에게 임신했는지 또는 임신을 했을 가능성이 있는지를 묻게됩니다.

검사 중

검사 중에는 불편함이 없습니다. 방사선 촬영은 누워서, 돌아누워서, 그리고 서 있는 상태에서 찍습니다.

검사 후

영상의학과 전문의가 방사선 영상기록을 판독한 후 주치의가 결과를 받고 당신과 결과에 대해 상의할 것입니다. 방사선 검사 동안에 당신에게 노출된 방사선은 다른 방사선 검사와 같이 즉시 당신의 몸을 통과할 것입니다.

로리와 함께하는 미국 문화 엿보기

내 생각엔 모든 병원이 더 좋은 환자복
으로 바꾸어야 한다고 생각해.
난 이 환자복이 너무 싫어.

이제야 왜 사람들이 ICU(다 보여)라고
하는지 알겠어.

주요구문

Step 1: ~부위에 방사선 촬영을 하겠습니다.

1. 흉부 방사선 촬영을 할 것입니다.
2. 복부 방사선 촬영을 할 것입니다.
3. 2장의 흉부 방사선 촬영을 할 것입니다.

Step 2: 검사가운

1. 옷을 벗고 병원 환자복으로 갈아입으세요.
2. 옷을 벗고 환자복의 여밈이 앞으로 오게 입으세요.

Step 3: 이쪽으로 오세요.

1. 이 보드 앞으로 와서 서 주세요
2. 이쪽으로 와서 보드를 향해 서 주세요.
3. 바로 여기에서 발바닥 그림을 밟고 이 보드를 보고 서 주세요.

Step 4: 자세 교정

1. 자세를 바로 하도록 도와드리겠습니다.

2. 방사선 촬영에 적절한 자세로 교정하기 위해 환자분의 신체에 손을 대겠습니다.
3. 뒤로 조금만 가 주시겠습니까?
4. 왼쪽 방향으로 조금만 가 주시겠어요?
5. 오른쪽 방향으로 반 걸음만 가세요.
6. 왼쪽 어깨를 조금만 내려 주시겠습니까?
7. 차렷 자세를 하세요.
8. 팔을 어깨 높이로 올리세요.
9. 얼굴을 이쪽 방향으로 돌리세요.
10. 신발을 벗고 방사선 촬영 테이블에 올라오세요.
11. 등을 대고 누우세요.
12. 머리는 이쪽에 다리는 저 아래쪽에 놓으세요.
13. 왼쪽 부위를 찍겠으니 오른쪽으로 돌아 누우세요

Step 5: 움직이지 마세요!

1. 방사선 촬영을 하는 동안 움직이지 마세요.
2. 그 자세를 유지하세요.
3. 이 상태로 잠시만 움직이지 마세요.

Step 6: 숨을 참아주세요!

1. 영상이 흔들리지 않게 몇 초 동안 숨을 참으세요.
2. 깊게 숨을 들이쉬고 참으세요.
3. 이제 숨을 깊게 들이쉬고 잠시 동안 숨을 참으세요.

Step 7: 숨 쉬세요.

1. 이제 숨을 쉬셔도 됩니다.
2. 숨을 내 쉬셔도 됩니다.

Step 8: 검사가 다 끝났나요?

1. 다 끝났나요?
2. 검사가 다 끝난 거죠?
3. 다 된 건가요?

Step 9: 옷 입으셔도 됩니다.

1. 영상을 확인한 후 곧바로 옷을 입으실 수 있습니다.,
2. 다 되었습니다. 영상이 나오면 곧 옷을 입을 수 있습니다.

2. Chest X-ray Examination

흉부 방사선 검사

독해구문

흉부 방사선 검사에 관하여

흉부 방사선

흉부 방사선 촬영은 소량의 방사선을 사용한 심장과 폐의 사진과 같은 영상입니다. 일반적으로 두 방향에서 촬영합니다. 한 방향은 등 뒤쪽에서 흉부로 방사선이 투과하는 전후 방향과, 다른 한 방향은 한 측면에서 다른 측면으로 방사선이 투과하여 흉부 영상을 촬영하는 측면 방향이 있습니다.

검사 중

검사실 안에서, 방사선사는 허리춤 뒤쪽에 방사선 차폐막을 놓아주거나, 또는 허리주위에 착용할 수 있는 짧은 차폐 앞치마를 건네줄 것입니다. 두꺼운 고무로 된 차폐는 생식기관을 방사선의 직접적인 노출로부터 보호해 줄 것입니다.

방사선사는 당신이 흉부높이에 설치되어 있는 방사선 촬영기 앞에 서 있으라고 지시할 것입니다. 손은 골반에 놓고, 어깨를 안쪽으로 구부리고 턱을 위로 들라고 지시할 것입니다.

그런 후에 방사선사는 깊게 숨을 들이 쉬고, 내 쉬고, 그리고 다시 한번 숨을 깊게 들이쉰 후 그 숨을 참으라고 지시할 것입니다. 폐의 모든 움직임이 방사선 영상을 흐리게 하기 때문에 숨을 참는 것은 중요합니다. 방사선사가 촬영을 한 후 숨을 쉴 때를 알려드릴 것입니다.

방사선사는 당신 흉부의 측면 또한 찍을 것입니다. 옆으로 돌고, 팔을 머리 위로 올린 자세를 유지하라는 지시사항을 들을 것입니다. 턱을 다시 들고 방사선 촬영을 하는 동안 숨을 참으세요. 방사선사는 추가적인 방사선 촬영이 필요한지의 여부를 알려드릴 것입니다.

나의 방사선 검사 이야기

흉부 방사선 검사

Receptionist: 무엇을 도와 드릴까요?

Patient: 예. 흉부 방사선 검사를 받으러 왔습니다.

Receptionist: 알겠습니다. 방사선 검사실로 가세요. 그러면 환자분의 이름이 곧 호명될 것입니다.

2분 후

Radiotechnologist: 안녕하세요. 제가 방사선사입니다. 안으로 들어오세요.

Patient: 감사합니다.

Radiotechnologist: 우선 몇 가지 확인할 것이 있습니다. 생년월일을 말씀해 주시겠습니까?

Patient: 1948년 8월 24일 입니다.

Radiotechnologist: 환자 팔찌를 보여주시겠습니까? 재차 확인을 하려고 합니다.

Patient: 물론입니다. 여기 있습니다.

Radiotechnologist: 감사합니다. 오늘 환자분의 주치의가 어떤 검사를 내렸는지 확인하겠습니다.

Patient: 알겠습니다.

1분 후

Radiotechnologist: 환자분의 주치의는 흉부방사선 검사를 지시하셨습니다. 우선, 병원가운으로 갈아입으세요. 저를 따라오세요. 이곳이 탈의실입니다. 질문사항이 있습니까?

Patient: 예. 제가 언더와이어브라(철사가 들어있는 브래지어)를 착용하고 흉부 방사선 검사를 받아도 되나요?

Radiotechnologist: 음, 흉부 방사선 촬영을 위해 브래지어를 벗으셔야 됩니다.

Patient: 알겠습니다.

Radiotechnologist: 또한, 모든 보석류 및 금속물질을 이 상자에 담으세요. 왜냐하면 금속 또는 단단한 물질들은 방사선 영상에 나올 수 있습니다. 이것은 오진을 야기시킬 수 있습니다.

Patient: 알겠습니다. 그러면 머리핀, 목걸이 및 휴대폰을 이 보관함에 넣겠습니다.

Radiotechnologist: 환자복으로 갈아입은 후에 옷과 보관함을 포함한 모든 소지품을 락커에 넣고 잠그세요. 그런 후 락커 열쇠를 제게 주세요.

5분 후

Patient: 열쇠 여기 있습니다.

Radiotechnologist: 예. 그러면 생식기관을 보호하기 위해 짧은 차폐 앞치마를 허리에 두르시겠습니다.

Patient: 알겠습니다.

Radiotechnologist: 이제, 흉부 방사선 영상 2장을 촬영하겠습니다.

보드 앞에 서 주시겠습니까?

Patient: 예.

Radiotechnologist: 보드 앞의 "발바닥 그림"을 밟고 서주세요.

발바닥 그림

Patient: 여기요?

Radiotechnologist: 네. 지시사항을 알려드리겠습니다. 먼저, 턱을 이곳에 대시고 손바닥이 위를 향하게 양손을 허리에 놓으세요.

Patient: 알겠습니다. 이렇게요?

Radiotechnologist: 아주 잘하셨습니다. 어깨를 앞쪽으로 당겨주세요. 숨을 깊이 들이 쉬시고 참으세요.

잠시 동안 그 자세를 유지하세요.

Patient: 네.

몇 초 후

Radiotechnologist: 숨을 쉬셔도 됩니다. 이제 2번째 영상을 촬영하겠습니다. 2번째 영상은 흉부의 측면에서 촬영하겠습니다. 촬영에 적합한 자세로 교정하기 위해 환자분의 신체에 손을 대겠습니다.

Patient: 알겠습니다.

Radiotechnologist: 보드에 흉부의 왼쪽측면을 대고 서서 팔을 머리 위로 올려주세요.

Patient: 알겠습니다.

Radiotechnologist: 그 자세를 유지하고 숨을 깊이 들이 쉬시고 참으세요.

몇 초 후

Radiotechnologist: 숨을 쉬세요. 영상을 확인하는 동안 밖에 나가셔서 잠시 기다려 주시겠습니까?

Patient: 네.

Radiotechnologist: 죄송하지만, 영상이 흔들렸기 때문에 촬영을 다시 해야 합니다.

Patient: 오우, 알겠습니다.

재 촬영. 3분 후

Radiotechnologist: 촬영이 잘 되었습니다. 검사가 다 끝났습니다. 여기 열쇠가 있습니다. 옷을 갈아입으세요. 그 후에 담당선생님의 진료실로 다시 가세요. 주치의가 검사결과를 알려줄 것입니다.

Patient: 알겠습니다. 감사합니다.

Radiotechnologist: 내원해주셔서 감사합니다.

3. Abdominal X-ray Exam
복부 방사선 검사

독해구문

복부 방사선 검사에 관하여

복부 방사선 검사

복부 방사선 검사는 비장, 위 및 장을 포함한 복부 부위의 장기들과 구조를 검사하기 위한 영상의학 검사입니다.

검사 중

검사는 병원의 영상의학과 또는 클리닉의 방사선사에 의해 촬영됩니다. 방사선 영상 촬영 테이블 위에 등을 대고 누우세요. 방사선 촬영기는 복부 부위 위에 설치되어 있습니다. 방사선을 촬영할 때 영상이 흐려지지 않기 위해 숨을 참아야 합니다. 추가적인 영상을 위하여 자세를 옆으로 바꾸거나 또는 일어서야 합니다.

주의사항

만일 지난 4일 이내에 비스무스를 함유한 펩토비스몰과 같은 약을 복용하셨다면, 의료진에게 말씀하세요. 이런 종류의 약은 검사에 지장을 줄 수도 있습니다.

나의 방사선검사 이야기

복부 방사선 검사

Patient: 복부 방사선 검사는 얼마나 걸리나요?

Radiotechnologist: 사실, 10분이 채 안 걸려요. 두 장을 촬영해야 합니다.

Patient: 알겠습니다. 그런데, 제가 환자복으로 갈아입어야 하나요?

Radiotechnologist: 네, 그렇습니다. 탈의실은 방사선 검사실 바로 옆방에 있습니다. 여기 환자복이요. 여밈이 앞쪽으로 향하게 병원가운으로 갈아입으세요.

Patient: 알겠습니다.

Radiotechnologist: 또한, 금속성 보석류, 휴대전화 및 허리 벨트를 락커에 넣어 주세요. 왜냐하면 그것들은 복부의 장기를 가릴 수 있습니다. 개인 소지품과 옷을 락커에 넣은 후, 잠그고 그 열쇠를 제게 주세요.

5분 후

Patient: 여기 있습니다.

Radiotechnologist: 네. 신발을 벗고 방사선 영상 촬영 테이블에 올라와 등을 대고 누우시겠습니까?

Patient: 바로 여기요?

Radiotechnologist: 예. 머리는 이쪽 위에 다리는 저쪽 아래에 놓으세요. 검사에 적합한 자세로 교정해 드리겠습니다.

Patient: 알겠습니다.

Radiotechnologist: 방사선 촬영을 할 준비가 되었습니다. 만일 검사 중에 움직이거나 숨을 쉬면 영상이 잘못될 수 있습니다. 이 상태로 잠시만 계세요.

Patient: 알겠습니다.

Radiotechnologist: 숨 쉬지 마세요.

2-3 초 후

Radiotechnologist: 숨쉬세요. 두 번째 방사선 촬영을 하겠습니다. 이제 왼쪽 부위를 촬영하겠으니 오른쪽으로 돌아 누우시고 팔을 귀에 붙이세요.

Patient: 이렇게요?

Radiotechnologist: 맞습니다. 이 자세를 잠시 유지하시고 숨을 참으세요.

2-3 초 후

Radiotechnologist: 숨쉬세요. 검사가 모두 끝났습니다.

Patient: 시간이 많이 소요되지 않는군요.

Radiotechnologist: 네. 협조해 주셔서 감사합니다. 영상이 제대로 나왔는지 확인하는 동안 잠시 밖에서 기다려 주시겠습니까?

Patient: 네.

Radiotechnologist: 영상이 잘 나왔습니다. 옷을 갈아입으셔도 됩니다. 열쇠 여기 있습니다.

Patient: 알겠습니다.

5분 후

Radiotechnologist: 담당의사선생님의 진료실로 다시 가세요. 그러면 주치의가 환자분에게 검사 결과를 말씀해 줄 것입니다.

Patient: 알겠습니다. 감사합니다.

Chapter 9

Vital signs

활력징후

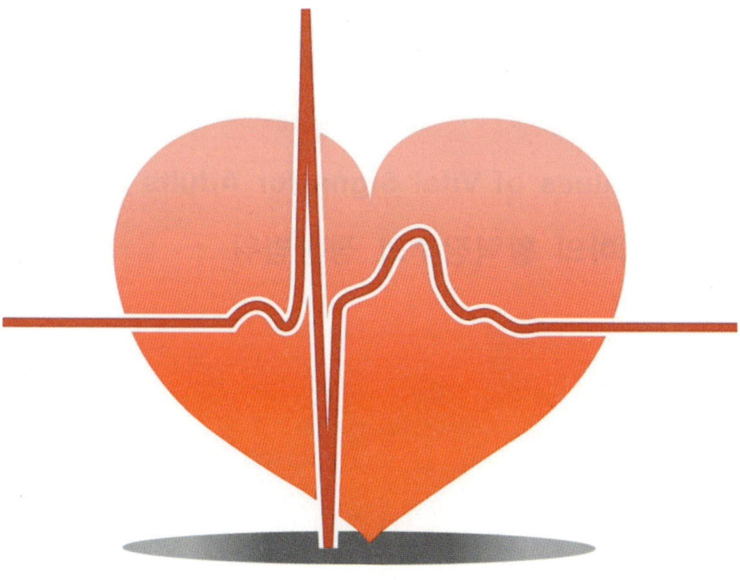

1. Vital Signs (V/S)
활력징후

- **What are Vital Signs?, 활력징후란?**
  - ■ Words, 어휘

- ***Code Breaker's Corner, 로리와 함께하는 미국 문화 엿보기***
  - ■ What is Fahrenheit?, 화씨란?
  - ■ Formula for Conversion between Fahrenheit and Celsius, 화씨와 섭씨간의 변환 공식

- **Normal Values of Vital Signs for Adults and Children, 성인과 소아의 활력징후의 정상범위**

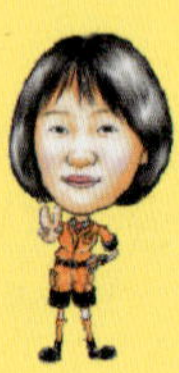

이 책의 녹음 파일은 www.ohgieun.com 에서 무료다운로드 하실 수 있습니다

Reading Material

What are Vital Signs?

Vital signs are measurable life signs. The term "vital signs" usually refers to the patient's temperature, pulse, blood pressure and respiratory rate. Vital signs are taken by health professionals and often vary by age.

Words

vital signs: 활력징후

temperature: 체온

pulse: 맥박

blood pressure: 혈압

respiratory rate: 호흡수

Code Breaker's Corner: 로리와 함께하는 미국 문화 엿보기

What is Fahrenheit?

The Fahrenheit is the unit of temperature used by most people in the United States in describing body temperature.

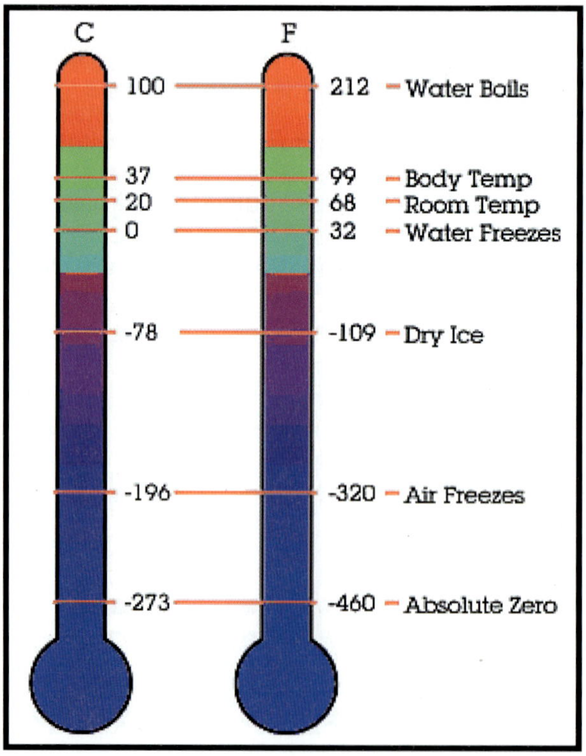

Formula for Conversion between Fahrenheit and Celsius

$$F = \frac{9}{5}C + 32 \qquad C = \frac{5}{9}(F - 32).$$

97.3F - 100.2F→ 36.3C - 37.9C

97.2F - 100.0F→ 36.2C - 37.8C

96.8F - 99.5F → 36.0C - 37.5C

97.7F - 99.5F → 36.5C - 37.5C

97.5F - 98.6F → 36.4C - 37.0C

97.0F - 99.0F → 36.1C - 37.2C

Words

Fahrenheit: 화씨

temp: (temp=temperature 를 줄여서 표기함) 온도

water boils: 물이 끓는다

room temp: 실내온도

water freezes: 물이 얼다

formula: 공식

conversion: 변환

Celsius: 섭씨

Normal Values of Vital Signs for Adults & Children

Adults:

Normal Temperature: Oral (96.8F - 99.5F),
Rectal (97.3F - 100.2F), Tympanic (97.2F - 100.0F)
Normal Pulse: 60 - 100
Normal Respirations: 12 - 20
Normal Blood Pressure: 100 - 139/60 - 89

Newborn:

Axillary Temperature: 97.7F - 99.5F
Pulse: 120 - 160
Respirations: 30 - 60
Blood Pressure: 73/55 systolic

One-year Old:

Axillary Temperature: 97.0F - 99.0F
Pulse: 90 - 130
Respirations: 20 - 40
Blood Pressure: 90/56 systolic

Toddler:

Axillary Temperature: 97.5F - 98.6F

Pulse: 80 - 120

Respirations: 20 - 30

Blood Pressure: 92/55 systolic

Pre-schooler:

Axillary Temperature: 97.5F - 98.6F

Pulse: 70 - 110

Respirations: 16 - 22

Blood Pressure: 95/57 systolic

School Age Child:

Oral Temperature: 97.5F - 98.6F

Pulse: 60 - 100

Respirations: 16 - 20

Blood Pressure: 107/64 systolic

Adolescent:

Oral Temperature: 97.5F - 98.6F

Pulse: 55 - 90

Respirations: 12 - 20

Blood Pressure: 121/70 systolic

Reference: Saunders Comprehensive Review for the NCLEX-RN Examination, 3rd edition, by Linda Anne Silvestri Reference: Expert 10-Minute Physical Examinations, 1997, Mosby's

2. Body Temperature (BT)
체온

- **Key Words, 주요어휘**
  - QUIZ: 내 단어장 점검하기
  - Drill: Word Search Puzzle, 연습문제: 어휘퍼즐
- **Key Expression for Taking Body Temperature, 체온관련 주요구문**
  - Words, 어휘
  - Drill, 연습문제
- **Reading Material: What is body temperature?, 독해구문: 체온이란?**
  - Words, 어휘
- **Method of Taking Body Temperature, 체온 재는 법**
  - Words, 어휘
- **Story of My Body Temperature, 나의 체온 이야기**
  - Dialogue: Taking a body temperature by ear, 대화: 고막체온 재기

■ Words, 어휘

■ Review, 복습

· **Story of My Body Temperature, 나의 체온 이야기**

■ Dialogue: Taking a baby's axillary temperature, 대화: 아기의 액와체온 재기

■ Words, 어휘

■ Review, 복습

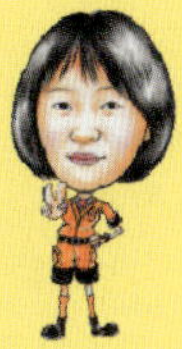

이 책의 녹음 파일은 www.ohgieun.com 에서 무료다운로드 하실 수 있습니다

Key Words

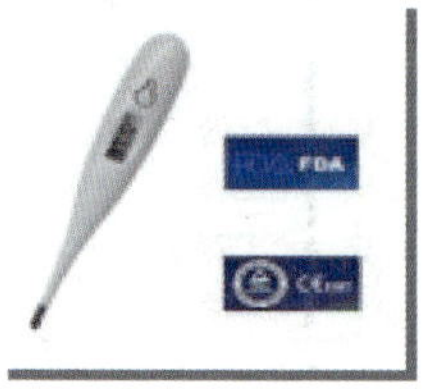

Electronic digital thermometer: 전자체온계

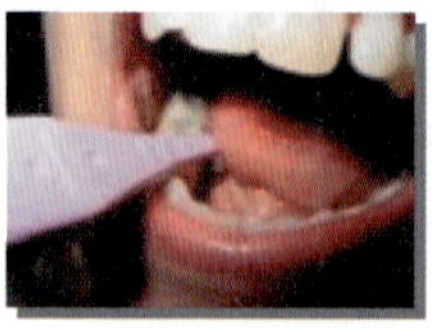

Oral thermometer: 구강체온계

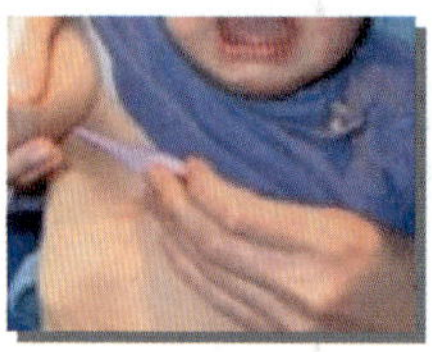

Axillary temperature: 액와체온

Armpit/Under arm: 겨드랑이

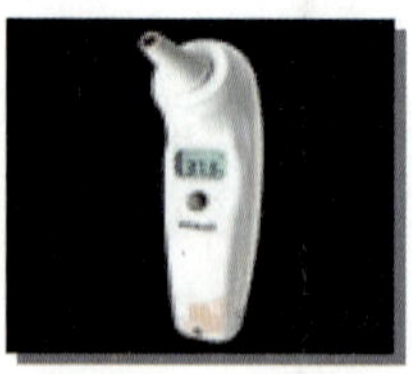

Ear thermometer: 고막체온계

Ear drum: 고막

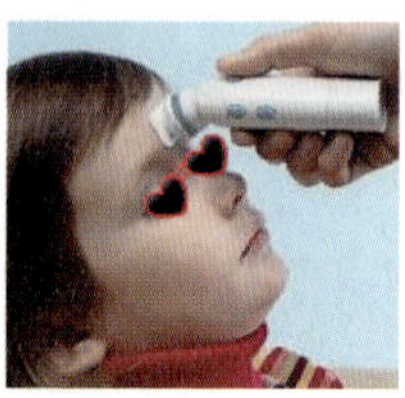

Forehead thermometer: 이마체온계

QUIZ: 내 단어장 점검하기 !!

아래 단어를 읽고 알맞은 뜻을 적어보세요.

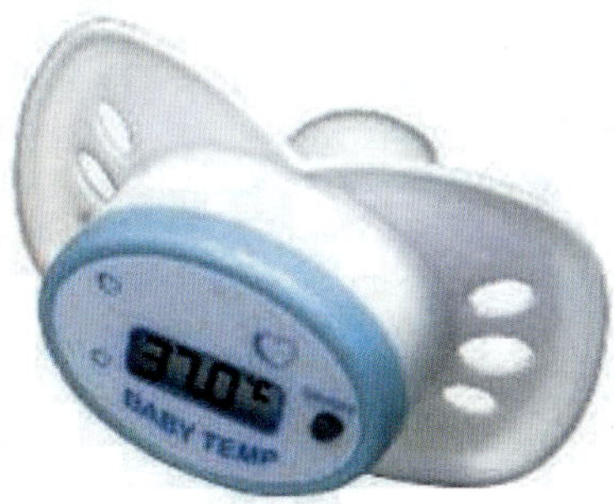

Oral thermometer: ....

Axillary temperature: ....

Armpit: ....

Under arm: ....

Electronic digital thermometer: ....

Ear thermometer: ....

Ear drum: ....

Forehead thermometer: ....

Drill: 아래의 단어를 ***Word Search Puzzle***에서 찾아보세요.

B	D	X	M	E	C	W	V	C	S	K	F	B	W	D	Q	A	M	V	N
P	V	I	S	Q	R	O	R	O	J	M	P	F	U	Y	H	X	N	J	R
D	V	U	Y	U	O	X	W	N	C	K	U	E	J	J	P	I	U	E	O
E	D	N	Q	T	M	M	M	I	G	O	X	U	Q	T	C	L	D	O	H
D	P	H	E	L	S	E	L	G	P	N	T	U	X	B	Q	L	R	M	D
V	K	R	A	O	H	F	R	I	S	H	O	T	N	M	C	A	S	W	N
Q	E	I	R	H	H	G	V	Y	T	L	V	L	C	E	L	R	W	N	K
N	E	K		L	T	K	K	E	J	E	L	O	Y		V	Y	L	E	O
D	F	B	T	N	R	H	K	F	V	D	O	K	T	D	A		T	G	V
G	I	M	H	I	W	C	W	R	K	I	B	H	F	R	P	T	P	O	W
F	O	R	E	H	E	A	D		T	H	E	R	M	O	M	E	T	E	R
T	M	Q	R	V	B	O	N	G	D	R	M	P	Y	X	U	M	A	A	K
D	L	U	M	Q	Q	A	W	B	M	L	I	X	N	B	W	P	Y	R	D
P	A	T	O	H	U	Q	Y	O	R	T	Q	J	P	A	Y	E	A		I
K	Q	E	M	I	X	Y	M	K	A	L	N	N	S	F	R	R	T	D	B
Y	A	S	E	O	R	E	W	C	S	V	P	V	N	E	J	A	M	R	B
S	C	V	T	L	T	F	A	B	K	G	W	I	A	A	J	T	P	U	V
W	M	I	E	E	K	R	X	R	N	I	L	Q	D	Y	K	U	H	M	O
T	E	F	R	G	I	W	O	N	P	J	R	N	Y	K	W	R	N	F	A
A	N	L	K	A	Q	Y	R	Q	I	E	G	F	H	Y	B	E	J	K	K

구강체온계, 액와체온, 고막체온계,

고막, 이마체온계, 겨드랑이

Key Expressions for Taking Body Temperature

Step 1

1. Let's take your temperature and see how it is.
2. I am going to take your temperature.
3. I am taking your temperature by ear.
4. I will do the axillary temperature.

Step 2

5. Would you please open your mouth and keep the thermometer under your tongue?
6. Open your mouth and say ahh, please.
7. Please turn your face this way.
8. Could you unbutton your shirt to take axillary temperature?

9. Now, I'll put the thermometer under your right arm.
10. Hold your arm down tightly at your side until the display light flashes on and beeps.
11. I will remove the thermometer when it makes the beeping sound.

Step 3

12. What is the normal body temperature?
13. What is my body temperature?
14. Your body temperature is 38°C (thirty-eight degrees Celsius).
15. It's 100.4°F (one hundred point four degrees Fahrenheit).
16. You have a fever of 105°F.
17. What is 38°C (thirty-eight degrees Celsius) in Fahrenheit?

Words

take your temperature: 체온을 재다

axiliary temperature: 액와체온

under your tongue: 혀 아래에

unbutton: 단추를 풀다

display light: 디스플레이어 불빛

flash: 불빛이 번쩍거리다

beep: "삐이" 하고 소리가 나다

normal body temperature: 정상체온

Celsius: 섭씨

Fahrenheit: 화씨

Helpful Tips

Temperature Converter: 온도 변환기

rounded results: 반올림결과

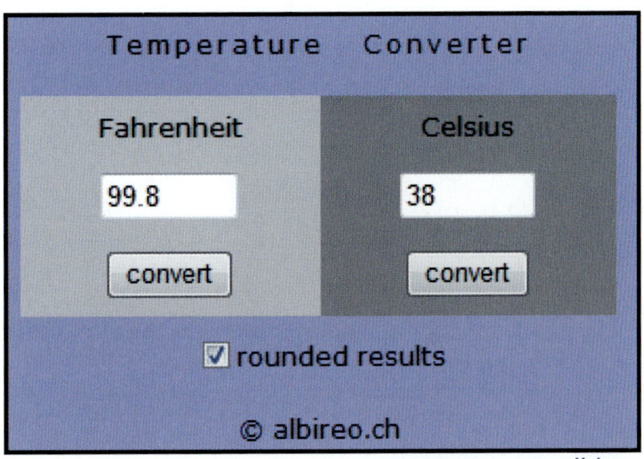

source: www.albireo

Drill: Q1-Q17을 영작하세요.

정답은 전 페이지의 Key Expressions for Taking Body Temperature를 참고하세요.

Q1. .... and see how it is.

채온을 재고 어떤 상태인지 보겠습니다

Q2. I am going ....

체온을 재겠습니다.

Q3. 고막체온을 재겠습니다. ....

Q4. 액와체온으로 재겠습니다. ....

Q5. 입을 벌리시고 혀 아래에 이 체온계를 넣으세요. ....

....

Q6. 아~하세요. ....

Q7. 얼굴을 이쪽으로 돌리세요. ....

Q8. 액와체온을 잴 수 있도록 셔츠의 단추를 풀어주시겠습니까? ....

....

Q9. 지금 체온계를 오른 팔 아래에 넣겠습니다. ....

....

Q10. .... until the display light flashes on and beeps. 디스플레이어 불빛이 번쩍거리고 "삐" 소리가 날 때까지 환자의 팔을 아래로 내려서 몸에 꼭 붙이세요.

Q11. I will ....when it makes the beeping sound.

제가 "삐" 소리가 나면 체온계를 빼겠습니다.

Q12. 정상체온은 몇도 인가요? ....

Q13. 제 체온은 얼마인가요? ....

Q14. 체온이 섭씨 38도입니다. ....

Q15. 체온이 화씨로 100.4도 입니다. ....

Q16. 체온이 화씨로 105도의 열이 있습니다..

Q17. 섭씨 38도는 화씨로는 얼마입니까? ....

....

Reading Material

What is body temperature?

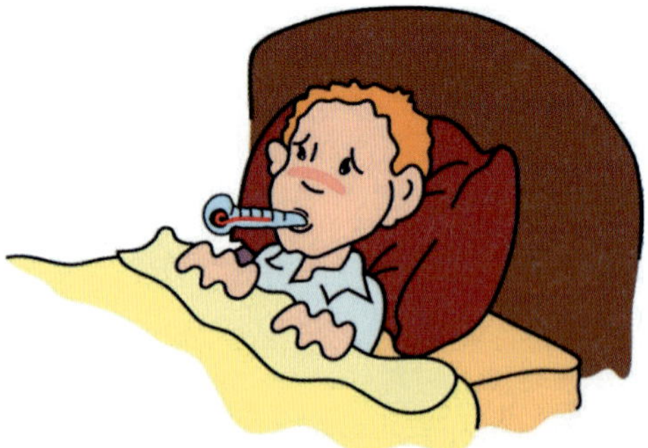

The normal body temperature of a person varies depending on gender, recent activity, food and fluid consumption, time of day, and in women, the stage of the menstrual cycle. Normal body temperature, according to the American Medical Association, can range from 97.8°F (equivalent to 36.5°C) to 99°F (equivalent to 37.2°C). Body temperature may be abnormal due to fever (high temperature) or hypothermia (low temperature). A fever is indicated when body temperature rises above 98.6°F(equivalent to 37°C) orally or 99.8°F(equivalent to 37.6°C) rectally, according to the American Medical Association. Hypothermia is defined as a drop in body temperature below 95°F (equivalent to 35.4°C).

Words

normal body temperature: 정상체온

gender: 성별

recent activity: 최근 활동

food and fluid consumption: 음식과 음료의 섭취

time of day: 하루 중 어느 시간

the stage of the menstrual cycle: 생리주기의 상태

Fahrenheit: 화씨

equivalent to: ~와 같다

Celsius: 섭씨

rectally: 직장으로

hypothermia: 저체온증

* Hypothermia is between 32-35°C.: 저체온증은 32-35°C 사이 입니다.

Methods of Taking Body Temperature

Orally

Temperatures can be taken by mouth using a digital thermometer to measure body temperature.

Rectally

Temperatures taken rectally tend to be 0.5 to 0.7°F (approximately 0.28 to 0.39°C) higher than when taken by mouth.

Axillary

Temperatures can be taken under the arm. Temperatures taken by this route tend to be 0.3 to 0.4°F (approximately 0.17 to 0.22°C) lower than those temperatures taken by mouth.

By ear

A special thermometer can quickly measure the temperature of the ear drum, which reflects the body's core temperature.

Words

orally: 경구, 입을 통하여

digital thermometer: 전자체온계

rectally: 직장을 통하여

axillary: 액와, 겨드랑이

under the arm/armpit: 겨드랑이

route: 경로

by ear: 귀를 통하여

ear drum/tympanic membrane: 고막

body's core temperature: 신체의 내부 온도

Story of My Body Temperature

Taking a body temperature by ear

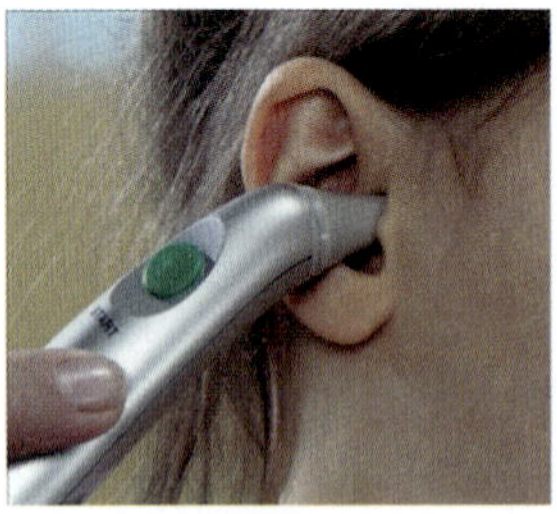

Nurse: What's your name?

Patient: Mark Anderson.

Nurse: What made you come in today?

Mr. Anderson: I've been suffering from a high fever for the past two days.

Nurse: Okay. Have a seat, please. I'm going to take your temperature by ear. Please turn your face this way.

Mr. Anderson: O.K.

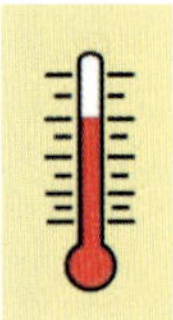

a few seconds later

Nurse: Your temperature is 38°C (thirty-eight degrees Celsius). You are running a high fever.

Mr. Anderson: What is 38°C (thirty-eight degrees Celsius) in Fahrenheit? I am still not used to degrees Celsius in Korea.

Nurse: It's 100.4°F (one hundred point four degrees Fahrenheit).

Mr. Anderson: Oh, I see.

Nurse: I will let your doctor know about the fever. Please wait in the waiting area.

Words

Celsius: 섭씨

run a high fever: 고열이 나는

Fahrenheit: 화씨

waiting area: 대기실

Review 각각의 구문을 영작하세요.
정답은 전 페이지의 Dialogue를 참고하세요.

Nurse: What's your name?

Patient: Mark Anderson.

Nurse: What made you come in today?

Mr. Anderson: 지난 2틀 동안 열이 나서 고생하고 있습니다.

....

Nurse: Okay. Have a seat, please.

고막체온을 재겠습니다. ....

얼굴을 이쪽으로 돌리세요. ....

Mr. Anderson: O.K.

a few seconds later

Nurse: 체온이 섭씨 38도입니다. ....

열이 높습니다. ....

Mr. Anderson: 섭씨 38도는 화씨로는 얼마입니까? ....

....

아직도 한국의 섭씨단위가 익숙지 않습니다. ....

....

Nurse: 화씨로 100.4도 입니다. ....

Mr. Anderson: Oh, I see.

Nurse: 주치의에게 환자의 열에 관해 말씀 드리겠습니다. ....

....

Please wait in the waiting area.

Story of My Body Temperature

Taking a baby's axillary temperature

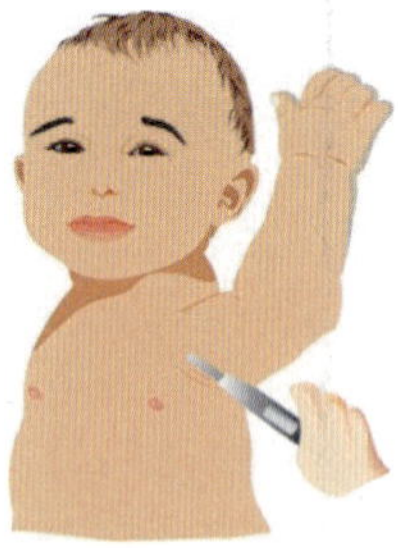

Nurse: Good morning, ma'am. What's your baby's name?

Ms. Smith: Jenny Smith.

Nurse: Thank you. I'd like to check your baby's temperature. I will do the axillary temperature.

Ms. Smith: Okay.

Nurse: I need to wash my hands first before taking her temperature. In the meantime, could you unbutton her shirt to take axillary temperature?

Ms. Smith: Sure.

Nurse: Now, I'll put the thermometer under her arm. Please hold her arm down tightly at her side until the display light flashes on and beeps.

Ms. Smith: I see.

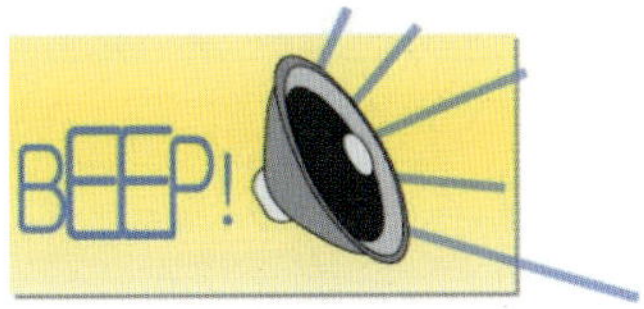

a few seconds later

Nurse: It's 38 degrees Celsius. Your baby is running a fever. I am going to report to the pediatrician now. You can button up her shirt.

Words

axillary temperature: 액와체온

unbutton: 단추를 풀다

Hold your arm down tightly at your side: 팔을 아래로 내려서 몸에 꼭 붙이세요.

flash on: 불빛이 들어오다

beep: "삐" 소리가 나다

pediatrician: 소아과 의사

button up: 단추를 채우다

Review 각각의 구문을 영작하세요.
정답은 전 페이지의 Dialogue를 참고하세요.

Nurse: Good morning ma'am.

아기의 이름이 무엇입니까? ....

Ms. Smith: Jenny Smith.

Nurse: Thank you.

아기의 체온을 재겠습니다. ....

액와체온으로 재겠습니다. ....

Ms. Smith: Okay.

Nurse: 체온을 재기 전에 먼저 제 손을 씻겠습니다. ....

....

그러는 동안 액와체온을 잴 수 있도록 아기의 셔츠 단추를 풀어 주시겠습니까? ....

....

Ms. Smith: Sure.

Nurse: 지금 체온계를 겨드랑이에 넣겠습니다. ....

....

불빛이 들어오고 "삐" 소리가 날 때까지 아기의 팔을 아래로 내려서 몸에 꼭 붙이세요. ....

....

Ms. Smith: I see.

a few seconds later

Nurse: 38도입니다. 열이 높군요. ....

....

소아과 선생님에게 알리겠습니다. ....

....

아기의 셔츠 단추를 채우셔도 됩니다. ....

....

3. Pulse Rate (PR)
맥박

- **Key Words, 주요어휘**
  - QUIZ: 내 단어장 점검하기
  - Drill: Word Search Puzzle, 연습문제: 어휘퍼즐
- **Key Expressions for Taking Pulse, 맥박관련 주요구문**
  - Words, 어휘
  - Drill: 연습문제
- **Reading Material: What is Pulse Rate?, 독해구문: 맥박 이란?**
  - Words, 어휘
- **Radial pulse, 요골맥박**
  - Words: 어휘
- **Story of My Pulse, 나의 맥박 이야기**
  - Dialogue: Radial Pulse, 대화: 요골맥박
  - Words, 어휘

- Review, 복습

· **Apical pulse, 심첨맥박**

- Words, 어휘

· **Story of My Pulse, 나의 맥박 이야기**

- Dialogue: Apical Pulse, 대화: 심첨맥박
- Words, 어휘
- Review, 복습

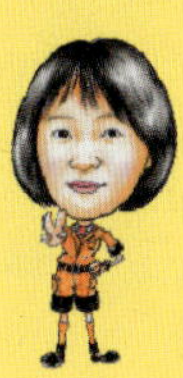

이 책의 녹음 파일은 www.ohgieun.com 에서
무료다운로드 하실 수 있습니다

Key Words

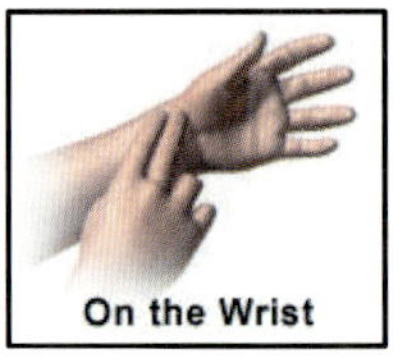

Radial pulse: 요골맥박

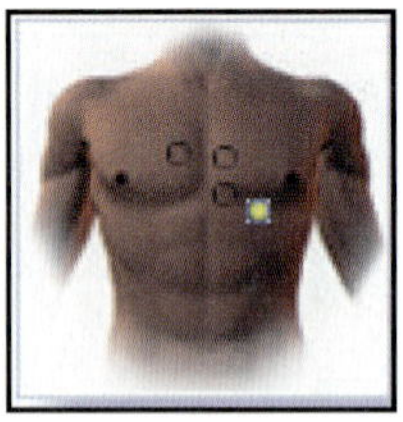

Apical pulse: 심첨맥박

Stethoscope: 청진기

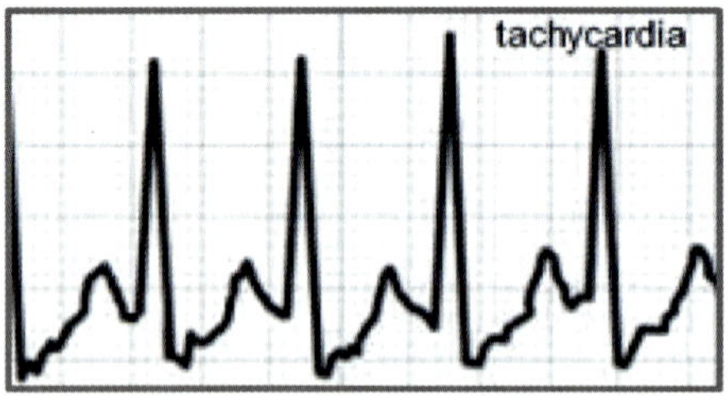

Tachycardia: 빈맥 100-120/min

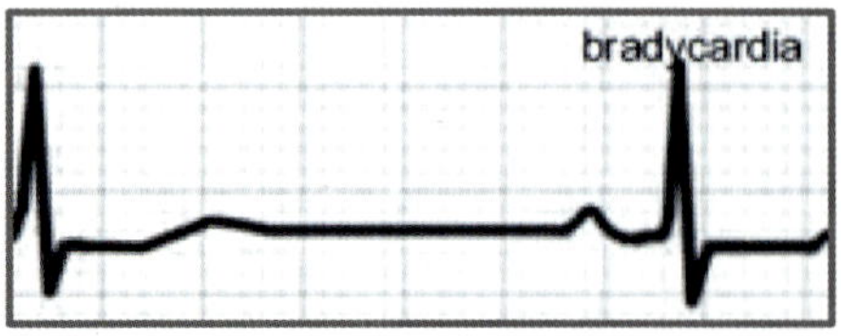

Bradycardia: 서맥 60 이하/min

Normal range: 정상맥박수치 80-100/min

QUIZ: 내 단어장 점검하기 !!

아래 단어를 읽고 알맞은 뜻을 적어보세요.

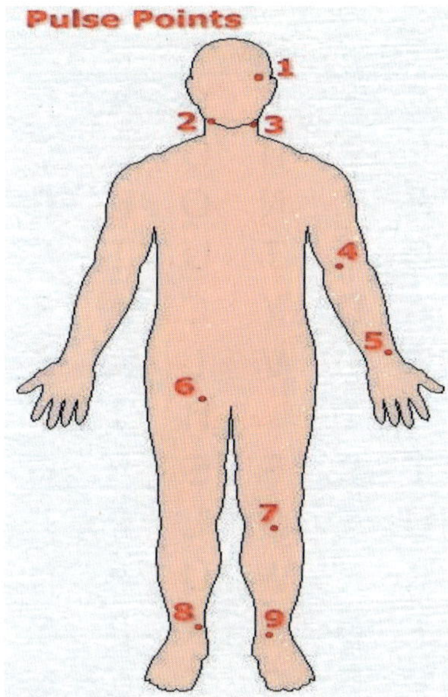

Radial pulse: ....

Apical pulse: ....

Tachycardia: ....

Normal range: ....

Bradycardia: ....

Stethoscope: ....

Drill: 아래의 단어를 ***Word Search Puzzle***에서 찾아보세요.

R	T	A	C	H	Y	C	A	R	D	I	A
A	S	T	E	T	H	O	S	C	O	P	E
D	L	N	R	T	N	Q	K	E	I	F	X
I	M	P	Q	Y	T	U	I	C	T	E	B
A	B	R	A	D	Y	C	A	R	D	I	A
L	V	X	T	I	V	L	W	J	S	X	Q
	E	H	U	I		H	J	Y	F	C	H
P	Y	A	T	P	F	S	R	G	O	L	L
U	P	K	U	J	S	L	F	F	M	F	I
L	N	L	K	N	W	U	P	N	A	Y	E
S	S	R	F	Q	N	R	B	Y	U	G	U
E	X	S	R	E	O	E	G	X	C	D	X

요골맥박, 심첨맥박, 빈맥, 서맥, 청진기

Key Expressions for Taking Pulse

1. I am going to take your pulse at your wrist.
2. I am going to listen to your apical pulse.
3. Please hold still while I am taking your pulse.
4. Please make yourself at home while I am listening to your heart.
5. Would you please give me your left arm?
6. Please unbutton your dress shirt so that I can listen to your heart.
7. Let me warm the stethoscope diaphragm using my hand first.
8. I am going to count your pulsations for one full minute.
9. I am counting your heartbeat for 60 seconds.

10. How's my pulse?

11. Is my pulse within the normal range?

12. Yours is 80 beats per minute.

13. It's very strong and regular.

14. Your heart sound is pretty good.

Words

take your pulse: 맥박을 재다

wrist: 손목

apical pulse: 심첨맥박

hold still: 움직이지 마세요

stethoscope: 청진기

diaphragm: (청진기의) 다이어프램

count your pulsations: 맥박수를 세다

one full minute: 60초 동안

within the normal range: 정상맥박수치

strong and regular: 힘차고 규칙적인

Drill: Q1-Q14를 영작하세요.

정답은 전 페이지의 Key Expressions를 참고하세요.

Q1. 손목에서 맥박을 재겠습니다. ....

Q2. 심장소리를 듣겠습니다. ....

Q3. Please hold still ....

제가 맥박을 재는 동안 움직이지 마세요.

Q4. Please make yourself at home ....

심장소리를 듣는 동안 긴장하지 마세요.

Q5. 왼쪽 팔을 주시겠습니까? ....

Q6. 심장소리를 들을 수 있도록 와이셔츠 단추를 풀어 주세요. ....

....

Q7. 먼저 청진기의 다이어프램을 손의 체열로 따뜻하게 하겠습니다. ......

....

Q8. 일분 동안 맥박수를 세겠습니다. ....

Q9. 60초 동안 심 박동수를 재겠습니다. ....

....

Q10. 제 맥박은 어떠한가요? ....

Q11. Is my pulse ....

제 맥박은 정상맥박 수치에 속하나요?

Q12. 맥박이 분당 80회입니다. ....

Q13. 매우 힘차고 규칙적입니다. ....

Q14. 심장소리는 정상입니다. ....

Reading Material

What is Pulse Rate?

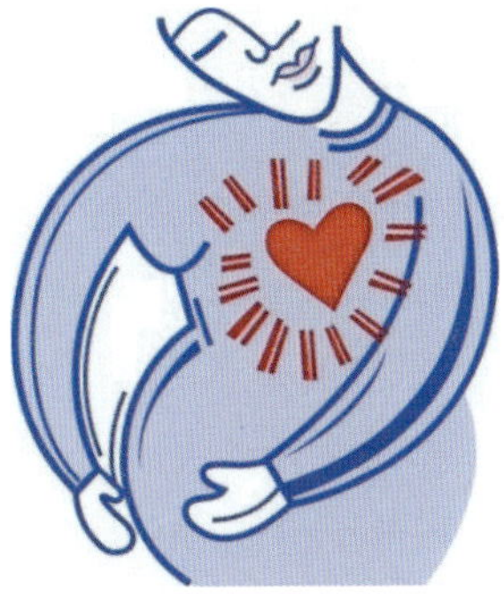

The pulse rate measures the number of heart beats per minute. As the heart pushes blood through the arteries, the arteries expand and contract with the flow of the blood. Taking a pulse not only measures the heart rate, but also indicates the following:

- heart rhythm
- strength of the pulse

The normal pulse for healthy adults ranges from 60 to 100 beats per minute. The pulse rate may fluctuate and increase with exercise, illness, injury, and emotions. Females 12 and older, in general, tend to have faster heart rates than do males. Athletes, such as runners, who do a lot of cardiovascular conditioning, may have heart rates near 40 beats per minute and experience no problems.

Words

artery: 동맥

expand: 확장

contract: 수축

the flow of the blood: 혈류의 흐름

heart rhythm: 심장의 리듬

strength of the pulse: 맥박의 세기

fluctuate: 변하다

illness: 질병

injury: 상해

emotions: 감정

female: 여성

athlete: 운동선수

cardiovascular: 심혈관계

Radial Pulse

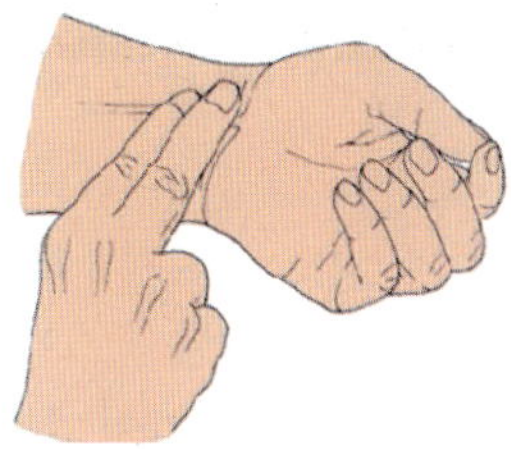

The radial pulse is taken over the radial artery in the wrist. The index and middle finger are used for this. You should not use a thumb as the thumb has a pulse as well and could give false readings.

Words

radial pulse: 요골맥박

radial artery: 요골동맥

as: 왜냐하면

thumb: 엄지

reading(s): 수치

Story of My Pulse

Radial pulse

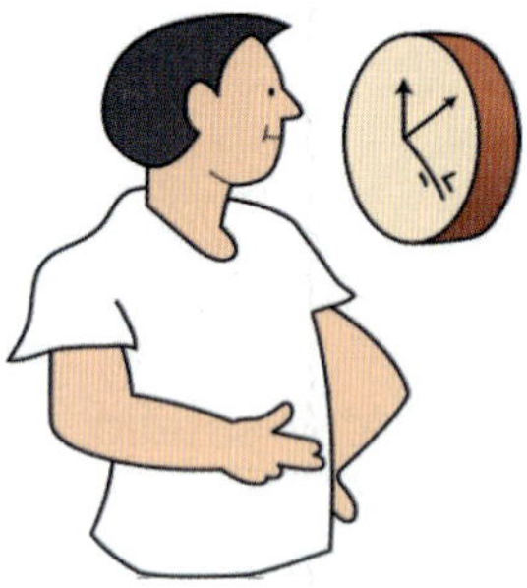

Nurse: Ms. Choi, I am going to take your pulse. Would you please give me your left arm?

Ms. Choi: Here it is.

Nurse: I will place the index and middle finger over the underside of the wrist, below the base of the thumb. Then, I will press firmly with flat fingers until I feel the pulse. There is a slight pressure from my fingers. I am going to count your pulsations for one full minute.

Ms. Choi: I see.

Nurse: Please hold still while I am taking your pulse.

Ms. Choi: O.K.

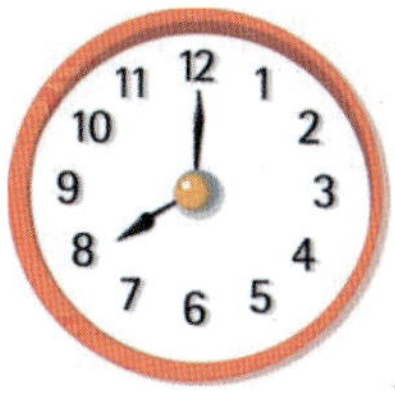

1 minute later

Nurse: We are all finished.

Ms. Choi: How's my pulse?

Nurse: Yours is very strong and regular. It's 80 beats per minute. The normal range is between 80 to 100 beats per minute.

Ms. Choi: You mean my pulse is normal, right?

Nurse: That's right.

Words

index and middle finger: 검지와 중지

underside of the wrist: 팔목의 안쪽

the base of the thumb: 엄지손가락 기저부

the normal range: 정상범주

Review 각각의 구문을 영작하세요.
정답은 전 페이지의 Dialogue를 참고하세요.

Nurse: 최선생님, 맥박을 재겠습니다. ....

....

왼쪽 팔을 주시겠습니까? ....

Ms. Choi: Here it is.

Nurse: 제가 검지와 중지를 팔목 안쪽의 엄지손가락 기저부에 대겠습니다. ....

그리고, 제가 맥박을 느낄 때까지 손가락을 펴서 누르겠습니다.

....

제 손가락에서 가해지는 압력을 느낄 것입니다.

....

일분 동안 맥박수를 세겠습니다. ....

Ms. Choi: I see.

Nurse: 제가 맥박을 재는 동안 움직이지 마세요. ....

....

Ms. Choi: O.K.

1 minute later

Nurse: We are all finished.

Ms. Choi: 제 맥박은 어떠한가요? ....

Nurse: 매우 힘차고 규칙적입니다. ....

맥박이 분당 80회입니다. ....

정상맥박수치는 분당 80-100회입니다.

....

Ms. Choi: 제 맥박이 정상이란 뜻이죠, 그렇지요? ....

....

Nurse: That's right.

Apical Pulse

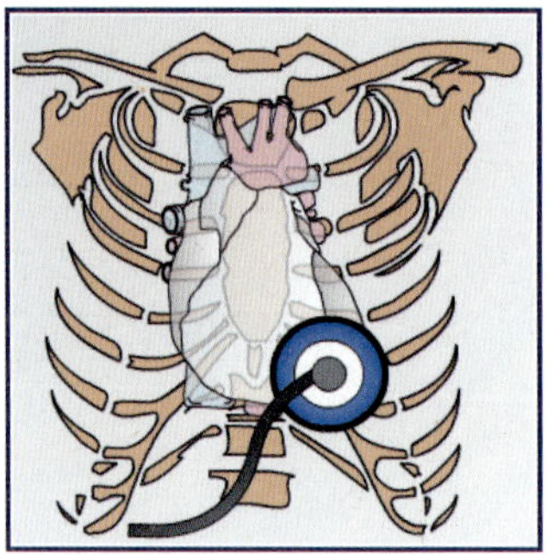

The apical pulse is a pulse that you take on the left side of the left nipple. You are taking the pulse which is the closest to your heart. Taking an apical pulse obtains more accurate pulse reading than can be counted at the radial site. Some patients who the doctor would request the medical assistance to obtain an apical pulse are:

· Patients with irregular heart rate

· Patients with bradycardia or tachycardia

· Patients taking cardiac medication

· Patients with faint radial pulse

Words

apical pulse: 심첨맥박

nipple: 유두

accurate: 정확한

pulse reading: 맥박수치

at the radial site: 요골동맥부위에서

irregular heart rate: 불규칙한 심 박동

bradycardia: 서맥

tachycardia: 빈맥

cardiac medication: 심장질환 약

faint radial pulse: 약한 요골맥박

Story of My Pulse

Apical Pulse

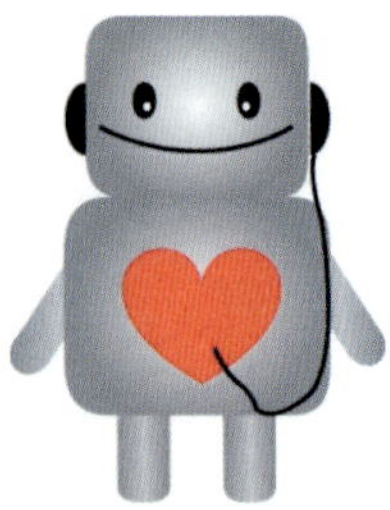

Dr. Gordon: Good morning, Mr. Kim.
How do you feel now?

Mr. Kim: I feel much better than yesterday.

Dr. Gordon: Good. By the way, did you experience any chest pain or sweating at night?

Mr. Kim: Not that I am aware of.

Dr. Gordon: Very good. Then, I am going to listen to your heart before you take your heart medication.

Mr. Kim: I see.

Dr. Gordon: Let me wash my hands first to put the stethoscope on you. Please unbutton your gown so that I can listen to your heart.

Mr. Kim: O.K.

Dr. Gordon: Now, I am ready. Let me warm the stethoscope diaphragm with my hands, so you won't feel cold.
Mr. Kim: Thank you, Dr. Gordon. You are so kind.

Dr. Gordon: My pleasure. It's warm enough. Please make yourself at home while I am listening to your heart.
Mr. Kim: Alright.

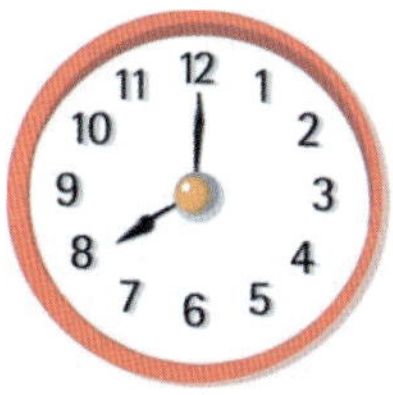

1 minute later

Dr. Gordon: I am all through now. You can button up your gown. Your heart sound is pretty good. You can take your heart medication now. I'll let your nurse bring your heart medication.
Mr. Kim: Thank you.

Nurse: Mr. Kim, I brought your heart medication. Here you are. You can take it now.
Mr. Kim: Okay.

Words

apical pulse: 심첨맥박

heart medication: 심장질환 약

stethoscope: 청진기

Helpful Tips

Anatomy of Stethoscope: 청진기 구조

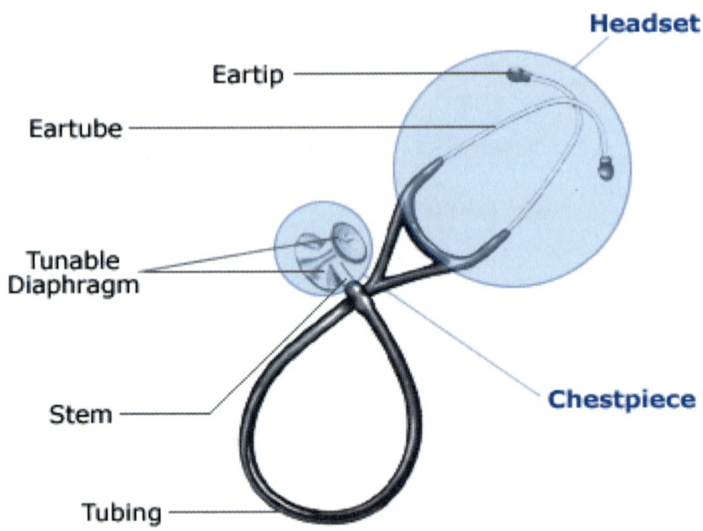

Headset: 헤드셋

Eartip: 귀꽂이

Eartube: 바이누랄

Chestpiece→Tunable Diaphram: **체스트 피스**→ 작은 원은 "벨", 큰 원은 "다이아프램"

Stem: 스템

Tubing: 연결관

Review 각각의 구문을 영작하세요.
정답은 전 페이지의 Dialogue를 참고하세요.

Dr. Gordon: Good morning, Mr. Kim. How do you feel now?

Mr. Kim: I feel much better than yesterday.

Dr. Gordon: 다행이군요. 그나저나, 밤에 흉통을 느끼거나 식은 땀을 흘렸나요? ....

....

Mr. Kim: Not that I am aware of.

Dr. Gordon: Very good.

심장약을 드시기 전에 심장소리를 듣겠습니다. ....

....

Mr. Kim: I see.

Dr. Gordon: 청진기를 대기 전에 제 손을 먼저 씻겠습니다. ....

....

심장소리를 들을 수 있도록 가운의 단추를 풀어 주세요. ....

....

Mr. Kim: O.K.

Dr. Gordon: Now, I am ready.

먼저 청진기 다이아프램을 제 손으로 따뜻하게 하겠습니다.

그러면 차갑지 않을 것입니다. ……………………………………………

……………………………………………………………………………

Mr. Kim: Thank you, Dr. Gordon. You are so kind.

Dr. Gordon: My pleasure. It's warm enough.

심장소리를 듣는 동안 긴장하지 마세요. ……………………………

……………………………………………………………………………

Mr. Kim: Alright.

1 minute later

Dr. Gordon: I am all through now. You can button up your gown.

심장소리는 매우 정상입니다. 심장약을 복용해도 됩니다. ………

……………………………………………………………………………

I'll let your nurse bring your heart medication.

Mr. Kim: Thank you.

Nurse: Mr. Kim. I brought your heart medication. Here you are. You can take it now.

Mr. Kim: Okay.

4. Blood Pressure (BP)
혈압

- **Key Words, 주요어휘**
  - ■ QUIZ: 내 단어장 점검하기
  - ■ Drill: Word Search Puzzle, 연습문제: 어휘퍼즐
- **Reading Material: What is Blood Pressure?, 독해구문: 혈압이란?**
  - ■ Words, 어휘
- **Sphygmomanometer, 혈압계**
  - ■ Words, 어휘
- **Key Expressions for Taking Blood Pressure, 혈압관련 주요구문**
  - ■ Words, 어휘
  - ■ Drill, 연습문제
- **Tips for Having Your Blood Pressure Taken, 혈압을 잴 때 유용한 정보**
- **Story of My Blood Pressure, 나의 혈압 이야기**

- Dialogue: BP by Sphygmomanometer, 대화: 혈압계로 잰 혈압
- Words, 어휘
- Review, 복습

· **Story of My Blood Pressure, 나의 혈압 이야기**

- Dialogue: BP with an Automatic Blood Pressure Monitor, 대화: 전자동 혈압계로 잰 혈압
- Words, 어휘
- Review, 복습

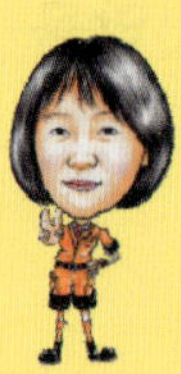

이 책의 녹음 파일은 www.ohgieun.com 에서
무료다운로드 하실 수 있습니다

Key Words

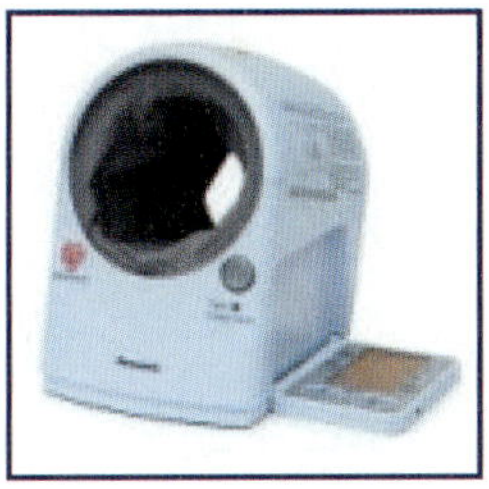

Tabletop blood pressure monitor/Automatic blood pressure monitor: 전자동 혈압계

Blood pressure: 혈압

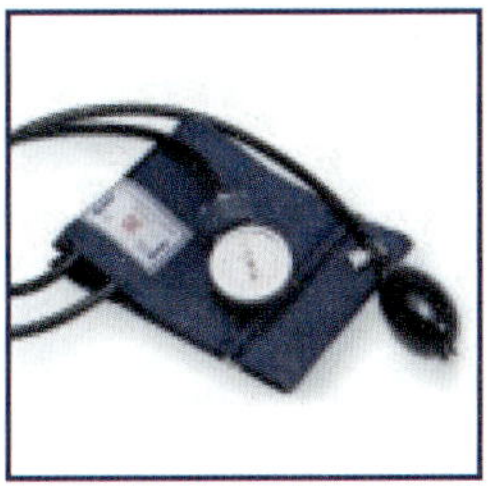

Sphygmomanometer: 혈압계

Blood pressure reading: 혈압수치

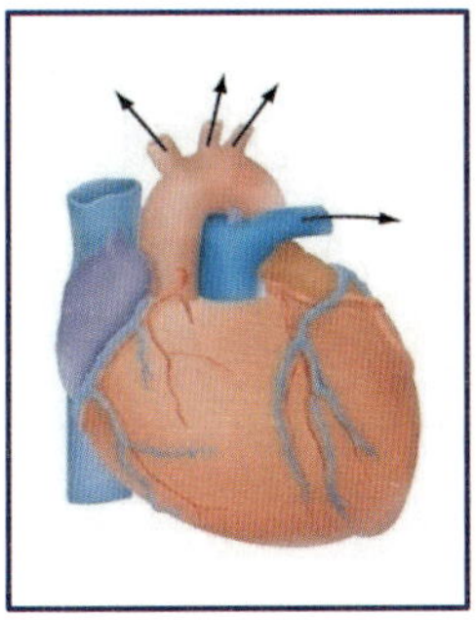

Systolic pressure: 수축기압

Artery: 동맥

Artery wall: 동맥벽

Hypertension: 고혈압

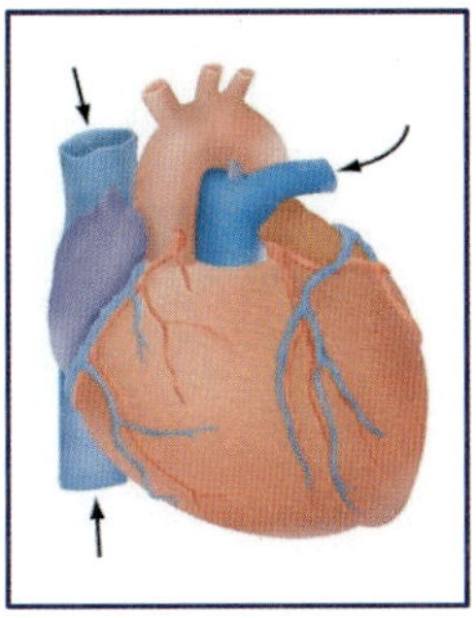

Diastolic pressure: 이완기압

QUIZ: 내 단어장 점검하기 !!

아래 단어를 읽고 알맞은 뜻을 적어보세요.

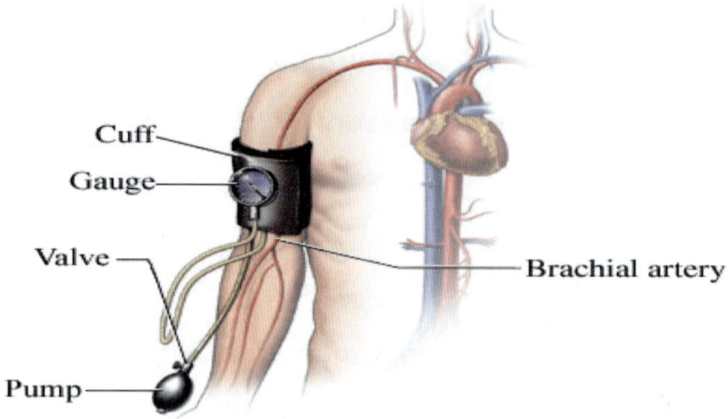

www.knowledgebase-script.com

Tabletop Blood Pressure Monitor/Automatic Blood Pressure Monitor: ....

Sphygmomanometer: ....

Systolic pressure: ....

Diastolic pressure: ....

Artery: ....

Artery wall: ....

Blood pressure: ....

Hypertension: ....

Blood pressure reading: ....

Drill: 아래의 단어를 ***Word Search Puzzle***에서 찾아보세요.

C	K	Y	N	P	D	I	H	N	I	U	E	L	W	X	T	A	F
J	V	I	K	M	I	X	W	Q	O	G	L	E	D	I	U	S	G
A	K	E	Q	A	A	C	J	S	Q	I	T	U	A	G	Y	I	O
K	V	N	I	J	S	M	T	P	O	V	K	X	R	S	Q	Q	S
L	U	K	G	N	T	B	T	Q	T	Q	S	Q	T	W	T	H	C
U	C	K	H	G	O	L	O	G	R	Q	Y	O	E	F	V	K	G
Y	J	B	H	A	L	O	C	W	W	L	L	X	R	N	B	J	B
Q	X	X	Y	Y	I	O	F	U	S	I	V	F	Y	F	F	C	J
B	L	S	P	K	C	D	B	X	C	X	W	P		D	N	X	A
R	K	O	E	T			X		I	U	I	X	W	T	E	H	Q
W	K	B	R	D	P	P	P	F	V	I	J	I	A	M	W	T	Y
K	K	B	T	T	R	R	T	H	J	U	N	C	L	E	G	A	P
H	B	B	E	R	E	E	R	N	C	R	S	B	L	E	N	V	Q
T	S	P	N	S	S	S	B	Y	Q	B	H	G	U	R	C	V	W
B	M	Q	S	P	S	S	N	H	C	Q	D	E	Y	H	O	C	T
T	P	U	I	Q	U	U	B	K	P	I	Q	A	B	M	K	J	F
F	R	U	O	A	R	R	K	E	O	N	X	N	G	N	X	P	I
E	D	X	N	K	E	E	A	U	K	G	O	J	M	O	I	G	H

수축기압, 이완기압, 혈압, 고혈압, 동맥벽

Reading Material

What is Blood Pressure?

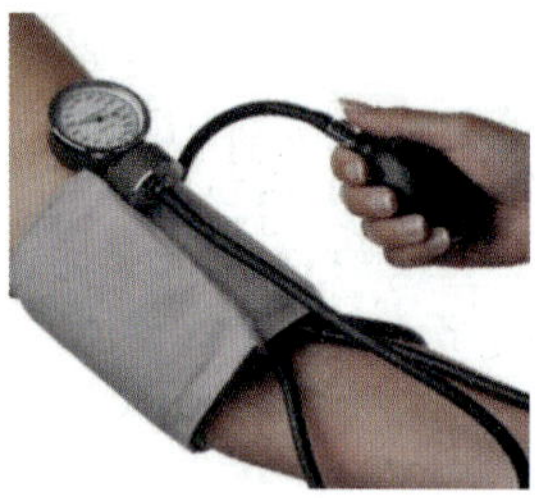

Blood pressure, measured with a blood pressure cuff and stethoscope by a nurse or other healthcare providers, is the force of the blood pushing against the artery walls. Each time the heart beats, it pumps blood into the arteries, resulting in the highest blood pressure as the heart contracts. Two numbers are recorded when measuring blood pressure. The higher number, or systolic pressure, refers to the pressure inside the artery when the heart contracts and pumps blood through the body. The lower number, or diastolic pressure, refers to the pressure inside the artery when the heart is at rest and is being filled with blood. Both the systolic and diastolic pressures are recorded as "mmHg" (millimeters of mercury). This recording represents how high the mercury column is raised by the pressure of the blood.

Words

blood pressure: 혈압

stethoscope: 청진기

healthcare provider: 의료진

against the artery walls: 동맥벽에 가해지는

artery: 동맥

contract: 수축

systolic pressure: 수축기압

diastolic pressure: 이완기압

mercury column: 수은 기둥

Sphygmomanometer

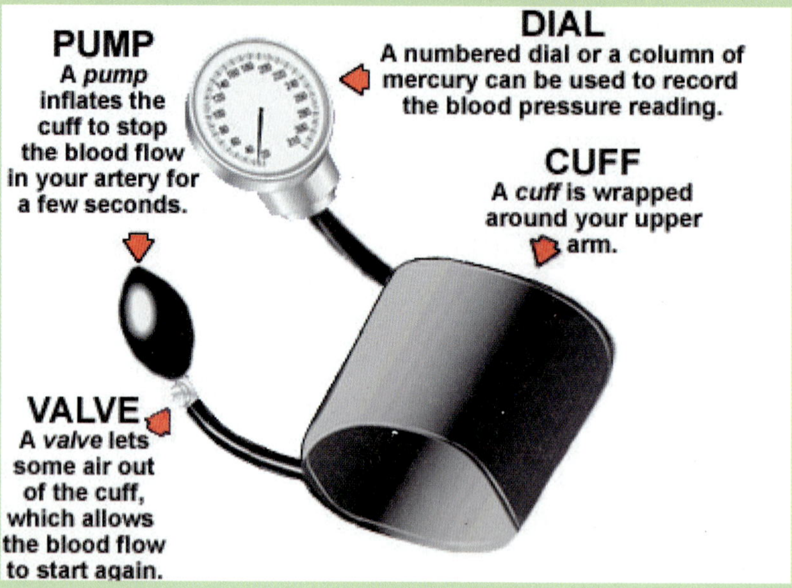

Resource: http:// www. nhlbi.nih.gov

Words

Sphygmomanometer: 혈압계

pump: 펌프

inflate: 부풀리다

cuff: 커프

blood flow: 혈류

numbered dial: 숫자가 쓰여진 다이얼

column of mercury: 수은 기둥

blood pressure reading: 혈압수치

valve: 밸브

Key Expressions for Taking Blood Pressure

1. Are there any precautions that I should take before measuring my blood pressure?

2. I am going to take your vital signs including your temperature and blood pressure.

3. I'd like to take your blood pressure.

4. I am going to check your blood pressure with this automatic blood pressure monitor.

5. Could you roll up your left sleeve?

6. I am going to put this cuff on your upper arm.

7. I will pump air into this cuff to get a reading.

8. Would you please put your left arm inside this cuff?

9. You will feel the pressure from the cuff on your arm while it is inflating.

10. You will temporarily feel numb and tingling in your hand.

11. I will put the stethoscope on your elbow crease.

12. The cuff will tighten up your arm and then slowly gets loose.

13. What are the normal values?

14. What should my blood pressure be according to my age?

15. Is my blood pressure normal?

16. What do the numbers mean?

17. It's 120 over 80.

18. Your blood pressure is very high.

19. Do you remember the result of your last blood pressure test?

20. When was the last time you had your blood pressure checked?

Words

precautions: 주의사항

take your vital signs: 활력징후를 재다

take your blood pressure: 혈압을 재다

put this cuff on~: ~에 이 커프를 감다

pump air into~: ~에 공기를 주입하다

temporarily: 일시적으로

numb: 감각이 무뎌지는

tingling: 저릿저릿함

elbow crease: 팔꿈치 안쪽의 접히는 부분에

tighten up: 조이다

get loose: 느슨해지다

normal values: 정상 수치

Drill: Q1-Q20을 영작하세요.

정답은 전 페이지의 Key Expressions for Taking Blood Pressure를 참고하세요.

Q1. ____________________

before measuring my blood pressure? 혈압을 재기 전에 지켜야 할 주의사항이 있나요?

Q2. 체온과 혈압을 포함한 활력징후를 재겠습니다. ____________________

____

Q3. 혈압을 재겠습니다. ____________________

Q4. I am going to check your blood pressure ____________________.

전자동혈압계로 혈압을 재겠습니다.

Q5. 왼쪽 소매를 걷어 주시겠습니까? ____________________

____

Q6. 이 커프를 상완(팔뚝)에 감겠습니다. ____________________

____

Q7. 혈압수치를 재기 위해 커프에 공기를 주입할 것입니다. ....

....

Q8. 이 커프 안에 왼쪽 팔을 넣어주시겠습니까? ....

....

Q9. 커프가 부풀어질 때 압력을 상완(팔뚝)에서 느낄 것입니다. ....

....

Q10. You will temporarily feel ....in your hand.

손에 일시적으로 감각이 무뎌지거나 저릿저릿함을 느낄 것입니다.

Q11. I will put the stethoscope ....

청진기를 팔꿈치 안쪽의 접히는 부분에 대겠습니다.

Q12. 커프가 팔을 조인 후 서서히 느슨해질 것입니다. ....

....

Q13. 정상 혈압수치는 얼마인가요? ....

Q14. What should my blood pressure be ....

제 나이에 적절한 혈압수치는 얼마인가요?

Q15. 내 혈압이 정상인가요? ……………………………………………………

Q16. 두 숫자는 무엇을 의미하지요? ……………………………………………

Q17. 혈압은 120에 80입니다. ……………………………………………………

Q18. 혈압이 매우 높습니다. ……………………………………………………

Q19. 마지막으로 잰 혈압수치가 얼마인지 기억하나요? ……………………
……………………………………………………………………………………

Q20. 마지막으로 혈압을 잰 게 언제입니까? …………………………………
……………………………………………………………………………………

Tips for Having Your Blood Pressure Taken

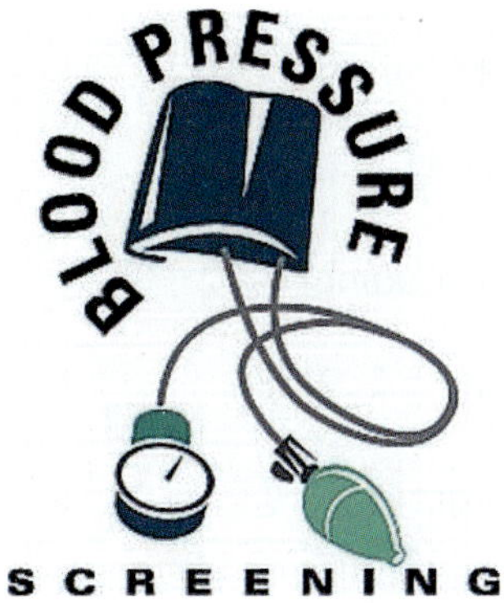

- Don't drink coffee or smoke cigarettes 30 minutes before having your blood pressure measured.
- Go to the bathroom prior to the reading.
- A full bladder can change your blood pressure reading.
- Before the test, sit for five minutes with your back supported and your feet flat on the ground.
- Rest your arm on a table at the level of your heart.
- Please don't talk while your blood pressure is measured.

Words

bathroom: 화장실

prior to the reading: 검사하기 전

a full bladder: 소변을 참으면

blood pressure reading: 혈압수치

back supported: 등을 기대고

feet flat on the ground: 발은 땅에 대고

at the level of your heart: 심장의 높이와 같게

Story of My Blood Pressure

BP by Sphygmomanometer

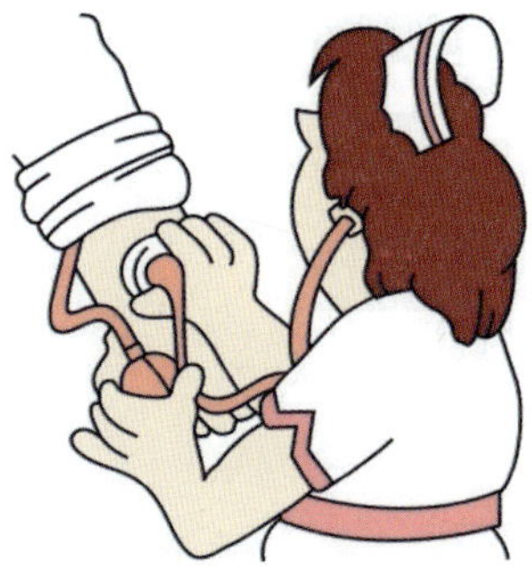

Nurse: How have you been feeling recently?

Lorri: I've been feeling a little light-headed.

Nurse: I see. Has anyone ever told you that you had high blood pressure?

Lorri: Not that I know of. I don't have any symptoms of high blood pressure at all.

Nurse: Usually people with high blood pressure have no symptoms, so we call it the silent killer. I am going to check your blood pressure. Would you please hold out your left arm and roll up your sleeve?

Lorri: Sure.

Nurse: Please relax your arm, and I will wrap the blood pressure cuff around your upper arm. It will be a little tight, and you will temporarily feel numb and tingling in your hand while it is inflating.

Lorri: Alright.

Nurse: Now, I will put the stethoscope on your elbow crease.

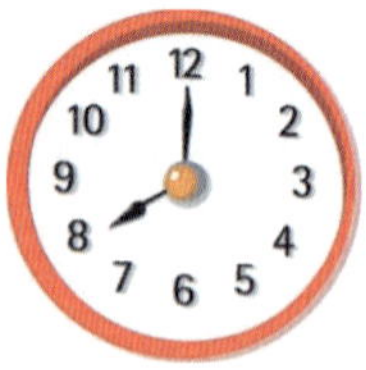

1 minute later

Nurse: Well, It's over now. Your blood pressure reading is one-twenty over eighty (120 over 80=120/80), which is fine.

Lorri: What does the reading tell you?

Nurse: The top number is the systolic blood pressure. This is the blood pressure when your heart is squeezing blood out. The bottom number is the diastolic blood pressure. It's the pressure when your heart is being filled with blood.

Lorri: Thank you for the explanation.

Nurse: No problem.

Words

light-headed: 어지러운

symptoms: 증상

silent killer: 침묵의 살인자

hold out your left arm: 왼팔을 내밀다

wrap: ~을 감다

temporarily: 일시적으로

numb: 무감각

tingling: 저릿저릿한

inflating: (공기를 주입해서) 부풀어지다

stethoscope: 청진기

elbow crease: 팔꿈치 안쪽의 접히는 부분

blood pressure reading: 혈압수치

systolic blood pressure: 수축기압

diastolic blood pressure: 확장기압

Review 각각의 구문을 영작하세요.
정답은 전 페이지의 Dialogue를 참고하세요.

Nurse: How have you been feeling recently?

Lorri: 어지럼증이 생겼어요. ....

Nurse: 알겠습니다. 고혈압이 있으십니까? ....

....

Lorri: 아니오. 고혈압증상이 전혀 없습니다. ....

....

Nurse: Usually people with high blood pressure have no symptoms, so we call it the silent killer.

혈압을 재겠습니다. ....

왼쪽 팔을 내미시고 소매를 걷어 주시겠습니까? ....

....

Lorri: Sure.

Nurse: 자, 팔을 편안하게 하세요. ....

이 커프를 상완(팔뚝)에 감겠습니다. ....

조금 조일 것입니다. 그리고 커프가 부풀어질 때 손에 일시적으로 감각이 무뎌지거나 저릿저릿한 감각을 느끼실 것입니다. ....

....

Lorri: Alright.

Nurse: 이제 청진기를 팔꿈치 안쪽의 접히는 부분에 대겠습니다.

1 minute later

Nurse: 끝났습니다. 혈압은 120/80입니다. 정상입니다.

Lorri: 두 숫자는 무엇을 의미하지요?

Nurse: 위의 숫자는 수축기압을 말합니다.

심장이 피를 심장 밖으로 뿜어낼 때 발생하는 압력입니다.

아래의 숫자는 확장기압입니다.

심장으로 혈액이 유입될 때 발생하는 압력입니다.

Lorri: Thank you for the explanation.

Nurse: No problem.

Story of My Blood Pressure

BP with an Automatic Blood Pressure Monitor

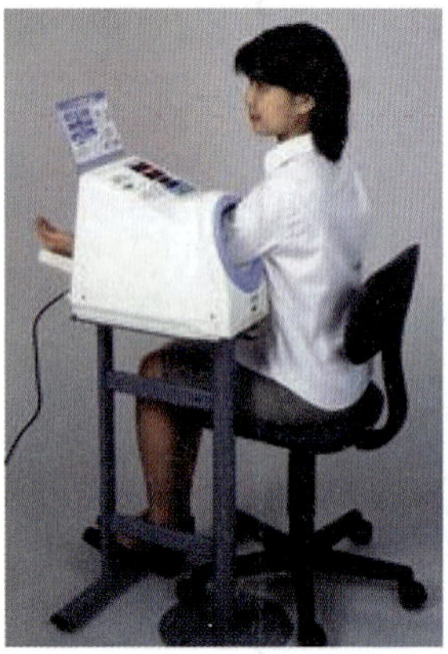

Nurse: Have you been having any problems lately?

Emily: Not really.

Nurse: Do you have a history of high blood pressure?

Emily: No. I have never been told that I have high blood pressure.

Nurse: That's good. Now, we are going to check your blood pressure with this automatic blood pressure monitor, and it will give us a reading.

Emily: Okay.

Nurse: I will give you some instructions for that. First, roll up your left sleeve and put your left arm inside this cuff, please. The cuff will tighten up your arm and then slowly gets loose.

Emily: Okay.

Nurse: Make yourself comfortable, please.

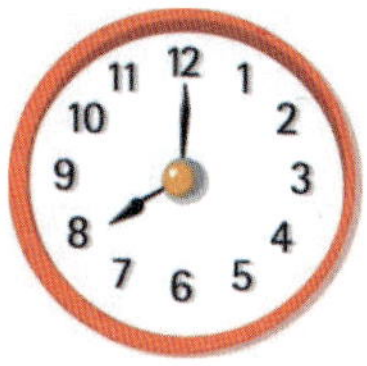

1 minute later

Nurse: It is all finished now. Your blood pressure reading is 150 over 100.

Emily: Well, is it possible for me to take it again because my blood pressure reading seems pretty high to me?

Nurse: Sure. You can take it again in 5 minutes. By the way, the blood pressure can fluctuate throughout the day.

Emily: Really? I didn't know that. Thank you for letting me know.

Words

an automatic blood pressure monitor: 전자동혈압계

high blood pressure: 고혈압

reading: 수치

instructions: 지시사항

roll up your sleeve: 소매를 걷다.

tighten up: 조이다

get loose: 느슨해지다

pretty: 매우

fluctuate throughout the day: 하루 24시간 동안 변하다.

Review 각각의 구문을 영작하세요.
정답은 전 페이지의 Dialogue를 참고하세요.

Nurse: 어디 불편하신 곳이 있습니까? ....

Emily: Not really.

Nurse: 고혈압증상이 있었던 적이 있습니까? ....

Emily: No. I have never been told that I have high blood pressure.

Nurse: That's good.

이제, 전자동혈압계로 혈압을 재겠습니다. 혈압수치를 알 수 있습니다. ....

....

Emily: Okay.

Nurse: 지시사항을 알려드리겠습니다. ....

먼저 왼쪽 소매를 걷어주세요. ....

그리고 커프 안에 왼쪽 팔을 넣어주세요. ....

커프가 팔을 조인 후 서서히 느슨해질 것입니다. ....

....

Emily: Okay.

Nurse: Make yourself comfortable, please.

1 minute later

Nurse: It is all finished now.

혈압은 150/100입니다. ....

Emily: 음, 혈압수치가 너무 높게 나온 것 같아서 그러는데 혹시 다시 잴 수 있을까요? ....

....

Nurse: 물론이지요. 5분 후에 다시 재시면 됩니다. ....

....

그리고, 사람의 혈압은 하루 24시간 동안 변할 수 있습니다. ....

....

Emily: Really? I didn't know that. Thank you for letting me know.

5. Respiratory Rate (RR)
호흡수

- **Key Words, 주요어휘**
  - QUIZ: 내 단어장 점검하기
  - Drill: Words Search Puzzle, 연습문제: 어휘퍼즐
- **Reading Material: What is Respiratory Rate? 독해구문: 호흡수란?**
  - Words, 어휘
- **Story of My Respiratory Rate, 나의 호흡수 이야기**
  - Dialogue: My Vital Signs, 대화: 나의 활력징후
  - Words, 어휘
  - Review, 복습
- **Words Review, 어휘복습**

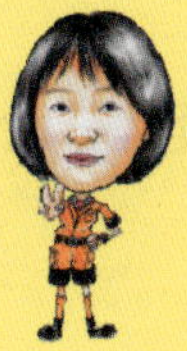

이 책의 녹음 파일은 www.ohgieun.com 에서 무료다운로드 하실 수 있습니다

Key Words

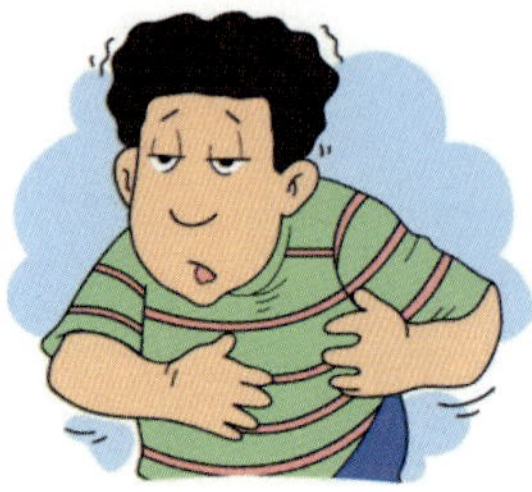

Respiratory rate: 호흡수

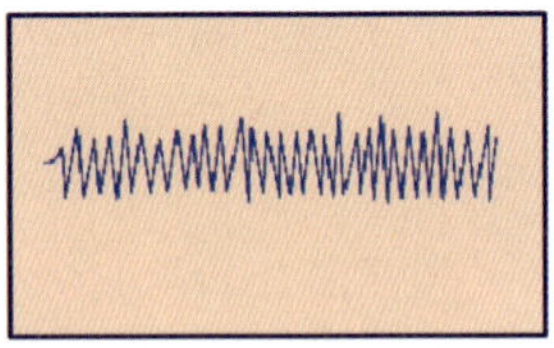

Normal respiratory rate: 정상호흡

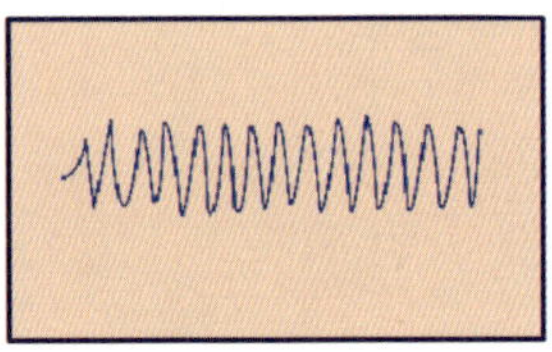

Bradypnea: 저호흡(느린호흡)

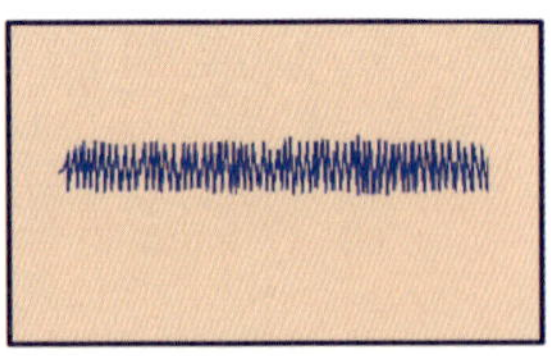

Tachypnea: 빈호흡(얕고 빠른호흡)

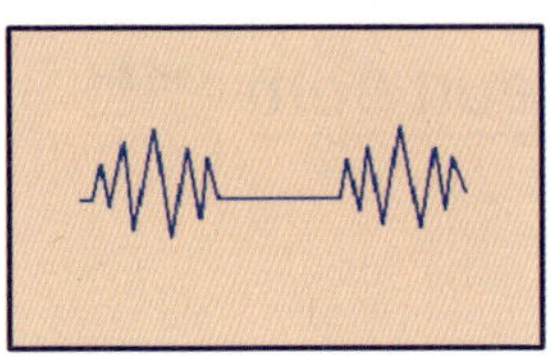

Apnea: 무호흡(간헐적으로 몇 초 동안 숨이 끊김)

QUIZ: 내 단어장 점검하기 !!

아래 단어를 읽고 알맞은 뜻을 적어보세요.

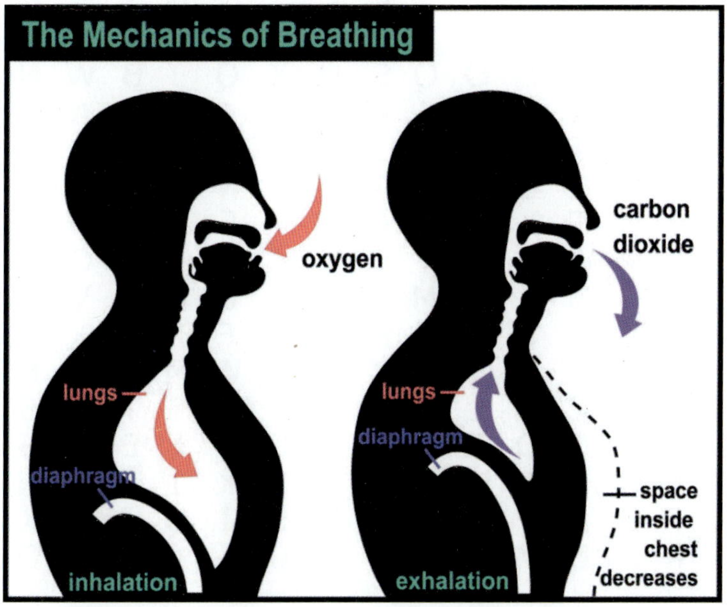

edb.utexas.edu

Respiratory rate:: ....

Normal respiratory rate: ....

Bradypnea: ....

Tachypnea:: ....

Apnea: ....

Drill: 아래의 단어를 ***Word Search Puzzle***에서 찾아보세요.

U	B	Q	D	O	M	I	R	K	J	G	G	J	M	V	G
Y	C	N	E	D	H	S	E	A	A	N	I	E	P	J	D
D	P	O	M	L	O	Q	S	U	X	Q	J	B	W	N	U
R	Y	Q	X	R	S	J	P	I	Y	A	X	E	A	M	P
B	G	C	I	K	F	U	I	D	F	P	M	O	P	P	L
J	N	M	S	C	U	A	R	O	H	N	I	D	P	G	U
W	J	B	T	X	B	U	A	J	Y	E	T	F	W	T	F
U	V	M	W	H	H	I	T	Y	A	A	P	D	G	E	S
Q	V	J	G	T	S	M	O	I	C	Q	N	C	V	A	H
T	F	L	X	L	L	H	R	H	U	F	X	E	X	E	T
M	M	Y	L	D	T	E	Y	R	S	W	M	G	W	H	H
W	G	Y	C	Y	L	P		W	E	R	I	T	F	S	P
L	K	P	G	O	N	N	R	L	O	Q	F	E	I	G	G
O	C	Q	L	E	W	D	A	K	K	K	I	J	X	N	Y
P	F	B	A	F	Q	V	T	H	E	I	U	Q	H	K	U
B	R	A	D	Y	P	N	E	A	U	I	V	I	H	D	D

호흡수, 저호흡(느린호흡),

무호흡(간헐적으로 몇 초 동안 숨이 끊김),

빈호흡(얕고 빠른호흡)

Reading Material

What is Respiratory Rate?

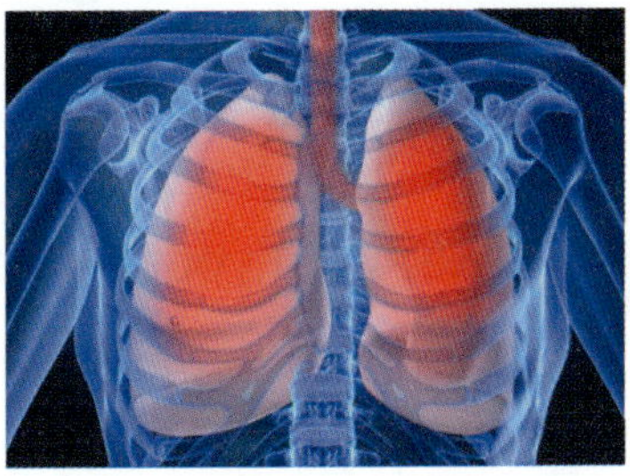

A respiratory rate, or breathing rate, is the number of breaths a person takes in 1 minute while at rest. Respiratory rate can be measured by counting the number of times a person's chest rises and falls within a minute. An individual's normal respiratory rate will change based on his or her age and an abnormally high or low respiratory rate may indicate certain medical conditions. The aim is to determine if the respirations are normal, abnormally fast (tachypnea), abnormally slow (bradypnea), or nonexistent (apnea).

Words

number of times: 횟수
tachypnea: 빈호흡
bradypnea: 저호흡
apnea: 무호흡

Story of My Respiratory Rate

My Vital Signs

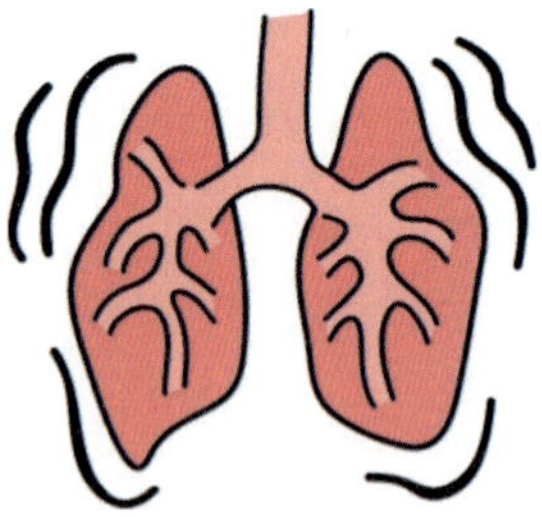

Nurse: I am your nurse today. How are you this morning?

Patient: Pretty good. Thanks.

Nurse: Let me verify a couple of things. What's your name and date of birth, please?

Patient: Jeffrey Johnson and 11/06/76.

Nurse: Thank you. Mr. Johnson, I am going to take your measurements first and then I'll check your vital signs.

Mr. Johnson: Alright.

Nurse: We use a scale with a stadiometer to measure your height (HT) and weight (WT).

Mr. Johnson: What is a stadiometer?

Nurse: Stadiometer is a vertical ruler with an arm that adjusts over your head. Would you please take off your shoes and stand on the platform?

Mr. Johnson: O.K.

Nurse: Your heels, buttocks, and shoulder blades should touch the measuring pole. Also, you need to look straight ahead, stand as tall as possible, and take a deep breath for the measurement. Let me check your position.

Mr. Johnson: Am I doing okay?

Nurse: Yes, you are. Now, the arm will get lowered and touch the top of your head and record your height and weight as well.

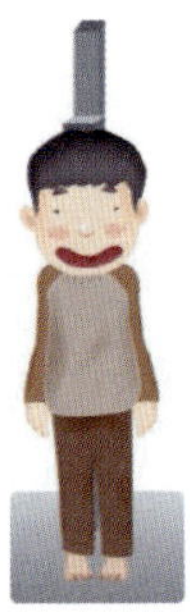

a couple of seconds later

Nurse: Please step off the platform and wear your shoes. You weigh 70 kilograms and you are 182 centimeters tall.

Mr. Johnson: I see.

Nurse: Now I will take your vital signs. Please have a seat on this chair.

Mr. Johnson: Right here?

Nurse: Yes. I'll take your temperature first. Please turn your face this way. It's 36.7C. Next I'll check your pulse. Could you give me your arm?

Mr. Johnson: Here you are.

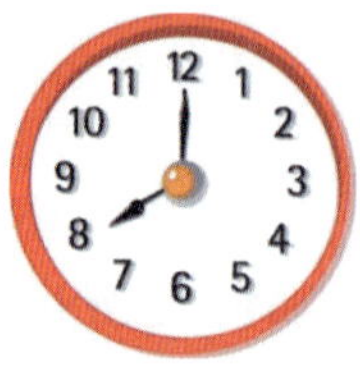

1 minute later

Nurse: Your pulse is 80 and your respiratory rate is 17. You are doing great so far.

Mr. Johnson: I didn't know that you measure my respiratory rate, too.

Nurse: When I check your pulse, I measure your respiratory rate as well.

Mr. Johnson: How do you measure the respiratory rate?

Nurse: Well, I usually count the patient's breathing for a minute by looking at the patient's chest. However, if the patient has normal respiratory rate, then I count the patient's breathing for 30 seconds and then multiply by 2.

Mr. Johnson: I see. Thank you for the explanation.

Nurse: No problem. Now I need to measure your blood pressure. Please roll up your sleeve for me.

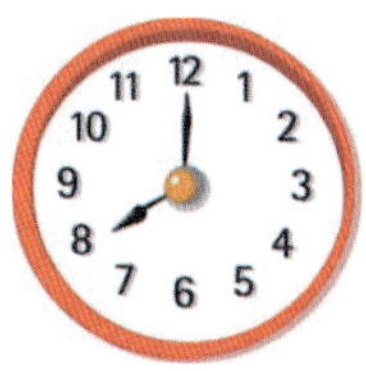

1 minute later

Nurse: It's 90 over 60.

Mr. Johnson: Is that too low?

Nurse: It's within the norm. Have you ever experienced light-headedness?

Mr. Johnson: No, not really.

Nurse: Then I wouldn't worry about it. Trust me. It's a lot better to have low blood pressure than higher one.

Words

take one's measurements: ~계측을 하겠다.

vital signs: 활력징후

scale: 저울

stadiometer: 신장계

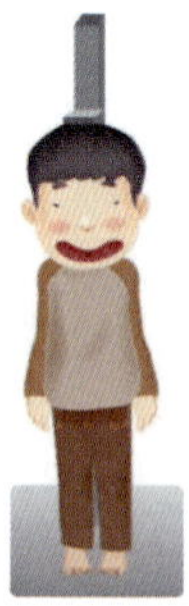

height: 키

weight: 몸무게

vertical: 세로의

ruler: (길이, 깊이, 키를 재는) 자

platform: (저울에 발을 딛고 서는) 저울 발판

heel: 발 뒷꿈치

buttocks: 엉덩이,

shoulder blade: 견갑골

multiply by: ~배로 하다

roll up your sleeve: 소매를 올리다

I experienced light-headedness (=I felt dizzy) 어지럼증을 느꼈어요.

Review 각각의 구문을 영작하세요.
정답은 전 페이지의 Dialogue를 참고하세요.

Nurse: I am your nurse today. How are you this morning?

Patient: Pretty good. Thanks.

Nurse: 몇 가지 확인하겠습니다. ....

....

이름과 생년월일을 말씀해주세요. ....

....

Patient: Jeffrey Johnson and 11/06/76.

Nurse: Thank you.

존슨선생님, 몸무게와 키를 먼저 재고 활력징후를 재겠습니다. .....

....

Mr. Johnson: Alright.

Nurse: 키와 몸무게를 재기 위해 신장계가 부착된 저울을 사용합니다. ....

Mr. Johnson: What is a stadiometer?

Nurse: 신장계는 환자의 머리 위에서 멈춰서는 측정막대가 부착되어있는 세로로 된 자 입니다. ....

신발을 벗고 여기 저울발판에 올라서세요. ....

....

Mr. Johnson: O.K.

Nurse: 뒷꿈치, 엉덩이와 견갑골(어깨뼈)이 측정대에 닿아야 합니다. ....

또한, 앞을 똑바로 보고, 가능한 한 키를 곧추세우고 숨을 들이쉬세요. ....

....

자세를 확인하겠습니다. ....

Mr. Johnson: Am I doing okay?

Nurse: 예. 측정막대가 내려와서 환자의 정수리부분에 닿을 겁니다. 그리고 키와 몸무게를 기록할 겁니다. ....

....

a couple of seconds later

Nurse: 저울에서 내려오셔서 신발을 신으세요. ....

....

몸무게는 70킬로그램이고 키는 182센티미터입니다. ....

....

Mr. Johnson: I see.

Nurse: 이제, 활력징후를 측정하겠습니다.

Please have a seat on the chair.

Mr. Johnson: Right here?

Nurse: 예. 체온을 먼저 재겠습니다.

이쪽을 보세요. 36.7C입니다.

이제 맥박을 재겠습니다.

팔을 주시겠습니까?

Mr. Johnson: Here you are.

1 minute later

Nurse: 맥박은 80이고 호흡수는 17입니다.

You are doing great so far.

Mr. Johnson: I didn't know that you measure my respiratory rate, too.

Nurse: 제가 맥박을 잴 때 호흡수도 잿습니다.

Mr. Johnson: 호흡수는 어떻게 재나요? ....

....

Nurse: 음. 환자의 흉부를 보며 1분 정도 호흡수를 셉니다.

....

그러나, 만일 환자가 정상적으로 호흡을 한다면 약 30초 정도 잰 환자의 호흡수에 곱하기 2를 합니다. ....

....

Mr. Johnson: I see. Thank you for the explanation.

Nurse: No problem.

혈압을 재겠습니다. ....

소매를 걷어 주세요. ....

1 minute later

Nurse: 혈압은 90에 60입니다. ....

Mr. Johnson: Is that too low?

Nurse: 정상범위에 있습니다. ....

어지러웠던 적이 있었나요? ....

Mr. Johnson: No, not really.

Nurse: Then I wouldn't worry about it. Trust me. It's a lot better to have low blood pressure than higher one.

Word Review: 위의 단어들을 복습하는 공간입니다.
정답은 Key Words를 참고하세요.

뜻: In English

전자 체온계: ....

구강체온계: ....

액와체온: ....

겨드랑이: ....

고막체온계: ....

고막: ....

이마체온계: ....

요골맥박: ....

심첨맥박: ....

청진기: ....

빈맥: ....

서맥: ....

정상맥박수치: ....

전자동 혈압계: ____________________

혈압: ____________________

혈압계: ____________________

혈압수치: ____________________

수축기압: ____________________

동맥: ____________________

동맥벽: ____________________

고혈압: ____________________

이완기압: ____________________

호흡수: ____________________

정상호흡: ____________________

저호흡(느린호흡): ____________________

빈호흡(얕고 빠른호흡): ____________________

무호흡(간헐적으로 몇 초 동안 숨이 끊김): ____________________

6. 해석 및 정답

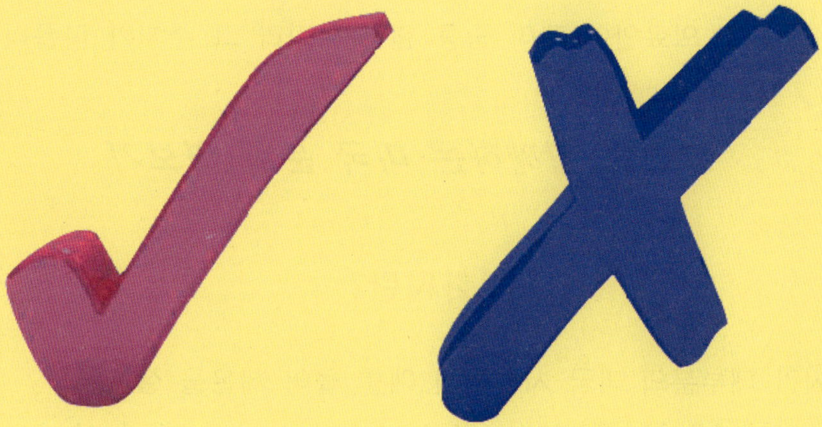

1. Vital Signs (VS)
활력징후

독해구문

활력징후란?

활력징후는 인간이 살아있는 상태를 측정한 것입니다. "활력징후"란 용어는 환자의 체온, 맥박, 혈압 및 호흡수를 의미합니다.

활력징후는 의료인이 재며 종종 연령에 따라 그 수치가 다릅니다.

로리와 함께하는 미국 문화 엿보기

화씨란?

화씨란 대부분의 미국 사람들이 예를 들어 체온을 잴 때 사용하는 온도의 단위 입니다.

성인과 아동의 활력징후 정상 수치

성인:

정상체온: 구강체온 96.8F - 99.5F → 36.0C - 37.5C

직장체온: 97.3F - 100.2F→ 36.3C - 37.9C

고막체온: 97.2F - 100.0F→ 36.2C - 37.8C

정상맥박수치: 60 - 100

정상호흡수치: 12 - 20

정상혈압수치: 100 - 139/60 - 89

신생아:

액와체온: 97.7F - 99.5F → 36.5C - 37.5C

정상맥박수치: 120 - 160

정상호흡수치: 30 - 60

혈압: 73/55 수축기압

만 1 세:

액와체온: 97.0F - 99.0F → 36.1C - 37.2C

정상맥박수치: 90 - 130

정상호흡수치: 20 - 40

혈압: 90/56 수축기압

만 1-3 세의 유아:

액와체온: 97.5F - 98.6F → 36.4C - 37.0C

정상맥박수치: 80 - 120

정상호흡수치: 20 - 30

혈압: 92/55 수축기압

<u>만 3-5 세:</u>

액와체온: 97.5F - 98.6F → 36.4C - 37.0C

정상맥박수치: 70 - 110

정상호흡수치: 16 - 22

혈압: 95/57 수축기압

<u>만 6-12 세:</u>

구강체온: 97.5F - 98.6F → 36.4C - 37.0C

정상맥박수치: 60 - 100

정상호흡수치: 16 - 20

혈압: 107/64 수축기압

<u>청소년:</u>

구강체온: 97.5F - 98.6F → 36.4C - 37.0C

정상맥박수치: 55 - 90

정상호흡수치: 12 - 20

혈압: 121/70 수축기압

2. Body Temperature (BT)
체온

어휘퍼즐 정답

B	D	X	M	E	C	W	V	C	S	K	F	B	W	D	Q	A	M	V	N
P	V	I	S	Q	R	O	R	O	J	M	P	F	U	Y	H	X	N	J	R
D	V	U	Y	U	O	X	W	N	C	K	U	E	J	J	P	I	U	E	O
E	D	N	Q	T	M	M	M	I	G	O	X	U	Q	T	C	L	D	O	H
D	P	H	E	L	S	E	L	G	P	N	T	U	X	B	Q	L	R	M	D
V	K	R	A	O	H	F	R	I	S	H	O	T	N	M	C	A	S	W	N
Q	E	I	R	H	H	G	V	Y	T	L	V	L	C	E	L	R	W	N	K
N	E	K		L	T	K	K	E	J	E	L	O	Y		V	Y	L	E	O
D	F	B	T	N	R	H	K	F	V	D	O	K	T	D	A		T	G	V
G	I	M	H	I	W	C	W	R	K	I	B	H	F	R	P	T	P	O	W
F	O	R	E	H	E	A	D		T	H	E	R	M	O	M	E	T	E	R
T	M	Q	R	V	B	O	N	G	D	R	M	P	Y	X	U	M	A	A	K
D	L	U	M	Q	Q	A	W	B	M	L	I	X	N	B	W	P	Y	R	D
P	A	T	O	H	U	Q	Y	O	R	T	Q	J	P	A	Y	E	A		I
K	Q	E	M	I	X	Y	M	K	A	L	N	N	S	F	R	R	T	D	B
Y	A	S	E	O	R	E	W	C	S	V	P	V	N	E	J	A	M	R	B
S	C	V	T	L	T	F	A	B	K	G	W	I	A	A	J	T	P	U	V
W	M	I	E	E	K	R	X	R	N	I	L	Q	D	Y	K	U	H	M	O
T	E	F	R	G	I	W	O	N	P	J	R	N	Y	K	W	R	N	F	A
A	N	L	K	A	Q	Y	R	Q	I	E	G	F	H	Y	B	E	J	K	K

Oral thermometer	Axillary temperature	Ear thermometer
Ear drum	Forehead thermometer	Armpit

체온관련 주요구문

Step 1

1. 채온을 재고 어떤 상태인지 보겠습니다.

2. 체온을 재겠습니다.

3. 고막체온을 재겠습니다.

4. 액와체온으로 재겠습니다.

Step 2

5. 입을 벌리시고 혀 아래에 이 체온계를 넣으세요.

6. 아~하세요.

7. 얼굴을 이쪽으로 돌리세요.

8. 액와체온을 잴 수 있도록 셔츠의 단추를 풀어주시겠습니까?

9. 지금 체온계를 오른 팔 아래에 넣겠습니다.

10. 디스플레이어 불빛이 번쩍거리고 "삐" 소리가 날 때까지 환자의 팔을 아래로 내려서 몸에 꼭 붙이세요.

11. 제가 "삐" 소리가 나면 체온계를 빼겠습니다.

Step 3

12. 정상체온은 몇도 인가요?

13. 제 체온은 얼마인가요?

14. 체온이 섭씨 38도입니다.

15. 체온이 화씨로 100.4도 입니다.

16. 체온이 화씨로 105도의 열이 있습니다.

17. 섭씨 38도는 화씨로는 얼마입니까?

독해구문

체온이란?

개인의 정상 체온은 성별, 최근의 활동, 섭취한 음식과 음료, 하루 중 어느 때인지, 그리고, 여성에게는 생리주기의 상태에 따라 다양합니다. 미국 의학 협회에 따르면 정상체온의 범위는 화씨로는 97.8°F-99°F 이며 섭씨로는 36.5°C-37.2°C 와 같습니다. 체온은 고열 또는 저체온으로 비정상적이 될 수 있습니다. 미국 의학 협회에 따르면 고열이란 체온이 구강으로 재었을 때 98.6°F(=37°C) 이상이거나 직장으로 재었을 때 99.8°F(=38°C) 이상인 경우를 의미합니다. 저체온증이란 체온이 95°F(35.4°C) 아래로 떨어진 경우를 의미합니다.

(저체온증은 32-35°C 사이 입니다.)

체온 재는 법

구강체온

체온은 전자체온계로 잴 수 있습니다.

직장체온

직장체온은 구강체온 보다 0.5 에서 0.7°F 더 높습니다.

액와체온

액와체온은 겨드랑이 부위에서 잽니다. 이 경로로 잰 체온은 구강으로 잰 체온 보다 0.3°F에서 0.4°F 더 낮습니다.

고막체온

특별한 체온계로 신체의 내부온도를 반영하는 고막체온을 측정할 수 있습니다.

나의 체온이야기

고막체온 재기

Nurse: 성함이 무엇입니까?

Patient: 마크 앤더슨입니다.

Nurse: 어디가 아픈가요?

Mr. Anderson: 지난 2틀 동안 열이 나서 고생하고 있습니다.

Nurse: 알겠습니다. 앉으세요. 고막체온을 재겠습니다. 얼굴을 이쪽으로 돌리세요.

Mr. Anderson: 네.

몇 초 후

Nurse: 체온이 섭씨 38도입니다. 열이 높습니다.

Mr. Anderson: 섭씨 38도는 화씨로는 얼마입니까? 아직도 한국의 섭씨단위가 익숙지 않습니다.

Nurse: 화씨로 100.4도 입니다.

Mr. Anderson: 오우, 알겠습니다.

Nurse: 주치의에게 환자의 열에 관해 말씀 드리겠습니다. 대기실에서 잠시 기다려주세요.

나의 체온 이야기

아기의 액와체온 재기

Nurse: 안녕하세요. 아기의 이름이 무엇입니까?

Ms. Smith: 제니 스미스 입니다.

Nurse: 감사합니다. 아기의 체온을 재겠습니다. 액와체온으로 재겠습니다.

Ms. Smith: 알겠습니다.

Nurse: 체온을 재기 전에 먼저 제 손을 씻겠습니다. 그러는 동안 액와체온을 잴 수 있도록 아기의 셔츠 단추를 풀어주시겠습니까?

Ms. Smith: 물론입니다.

Nurse: 지금 체온계를 겨드랑이에 넣겠습니다. 불빛이 들어오고 "삐" 소리가 날 때까지 아기의 팔을 아래로 내려서 몸에 꼭 붙이세요.

Ms. Smith: 알겠습니다.

몇 초 후

Nurse: 38도입니다. 열이 높군요. 소아과 선생님에게 알리겠습니다. 아기의 셔츠 단추를 채우셔도 됩니다.

3. Pulse Rate (PR)
맥박

어휘퍼즐정답

R	T	A	C	H	Y	C	A	R	D	I	A
A	S	T	E	T	H	O	S	C	O	P	E
D	L	N	R	T	N	Q	K	E	I	F	X
I	M	P	Q	Y	T	U	I	C	T	E	B
A	B	R	A	D	Y	C	A	R	D	I	A
L	V	X	T	I	V	L	W	J	S	X	Q
	E	H	U	I		H	J	Y	F	C	H
P	Y	A	T	P	F	S	R	G	O	L	L
U	P	K	U	J	S	L	F	F	M	F	I
L	N	L	K	N	W	U	P	N	A	Y	E
S	S	R	F	Q	N	R	B	Y	U	G	U
E	X	S	R	E	O	E	G	X	C	D	X

Radial pulse Apical pulse Tachycardia
Bradycardia Stethoscope

맥박관련 주요구문

1. 손목에서 맥박을 재겠습니다.
2. 심장소리를 듣겠습니다.
3. 재가 맥박을 재는 동안 움직이지 마세요.
4. 심장소리를 듣는 동안 긴장하지 마세요.
5. 왼쪽 팔을 주시겠습니까?
6. 심장소리를 들을 수 있도록 와이셔츠 단추를 풀어 주세요.
7. 먼저 청진기의 다이어프램을 손의 체열로 따뜻하게 하겠습니다.
8. 일분 동안 맥박수를 세겠습니다.
9. 60초 동안 심 박동수를 재겠습니다.
10. 제 맥박은 어떠한가요?
11. 제 맥박은 정상맥박 수치에 속하나요?
12. 맥박이 분당 80회입니다.
13. 매우 힘차고 규칙적입니다.
14. 심장소리는 정상입니다.

독해구문

맥박은 무엇입니까?

맥박은 일분에 심장이 뛰는 횟수를 측정한 것입니다. 심장이 동맥으로 혈액을 뿜을 때, 동맥은 혈류의 흐름으로 확장되고 수축됩니다.

맥박을 재는 것은 심박동률을 재는 것뿐만 아니라

- 심장의 리듬과
- 맥박의 세기도 알려 줍니다.

건강한 성인의 정상 맥박은 분 당 60-100회 입니다. 맥박은 변할 수 있고 운동, 질병, 상해와 감정에 의해 증가할 수 있습니다.

일반적으로 12세 이상의 여성은 남성들보다 심박동률이 더 빠릅니다. 심혈관계와 관계된 많은 운동을 하는 달리기선수와 같은 운동선수들은 분당 40회의 맥박을 가지고도 아무런 문제가 없습니다.

요골맥박

요골맥박은 손목의 요골동맥의 박동을 재는 것입니다. 맥박을 재는데 검지와 중지가 사용됩니다. 엄지를 사용해서는 안됩니다. 왜냐하면 엄지에서도 맥박을 느낄 수 있기에 맥박수가 잘못될 수 있습니다.

나의 맥박 이야기

맥박 재기

Nurse: 최선생님, 맥박을 재겠습니다. 왼쪽 팔을 주시겠습니까?

Ms. Choi: 여기 있습니다.

Nurse: 제가 검지와 중지를 팔목 안쪽의 엄지손가락 기저부에 대겠습니다. 그리고, 제가 맥박을 느낄 때까지 손가락을 펴서 누르겠습니다. 제 손가락에서 가해지는 압력을 느낄 것입니다. 일분 동안 맥박수를 세겠습니다.

Ms. Choi: 알겠습니다.

Nurse: 제가 맥박을 재는 동안 움직이지 마세요.

Ms. Choi: 알겠습니다.

1분 후

Nurse: 다 끝났습니다.

Ms. Choi: 제 맥박은 어떠한가요?

Nurse: 매우 힘차고 규칙적입니다. 맥박이 분당 80회입니다. 정상맥박수치는 분당 80-100회입니다.

Ms. Choi: 제 맥박이 정상이란 뜻이죠, 그렇지요?

Nurse: 맞습니다.

심첨맥박

심첨맥박은 왼쪽 유두의 왼쪽 부위에서 잰 맥박입니다. 심장에 가장 가까운 부위의 맥박을 잽니다. 심첨맥박을 재는 것은 요골부위를 재는 것보다 더 정확한 맥박수치를 얻을 수 있습니다. 때때로 의사는 심 박동이 불규칙적인 환자, 빈맥 또는 서맥인 환자, 심장질환 약을 복용하는 환자, 요골맥박이 약한 환자들의 심첨맥박을 잴 것을 요구합니다.

나의 맥박 이야기
심첨맥박 재기

Dr. Gordon: 안녕하세요, 김 선생님. 오늘은 좀 어떠세요?

Mr. Kim: 어제보다 훨씬 차도가 있습니다.

Dr. Gordon: 다행이군요. 그나저나, 밤에 흉통을 느끼거나 식은땀을 흘렸나요?

Mr. Kim: 아니요.

Dr. Gordon: 다행이군요. 심장약을 드시기 전에 심장소리(심첨맥박)를 듣겠습니다.

Mr. Kim: 알겠습니다.

Dr. Gordon: 청진기를 대기 전에 제 손을 먼저 씻겠습니다. 심장 소리를 들을 수 있도록 가운의 단추를 풀어 주세요.

Mr. Kim: 알겠습니다.

Dr. Gordon: 준비가 되었습니다. 먼저 청진기 다이아프램을 제 손으로 따뜻하게 하겠습니다. 그러면 차갑지 않을 것입니다.

Mr. Kim: 고맙습니다. 의사선생님께서는 매우 친절 하세요.

Dr. Gordon: 별말씀을요. 따뜻해졌습니다. 심장소리를 듣는 동안 긴장하지 마세요.

Mr. Kim: 네.

1분 후

Dr. Gordon: 다 끝났습니다. 가운의 단추를 채우셔도 됩니다. 심장소리는 매우 정상입니다. 심장약을 복용해도 됩니다. 간호사에게 약을 가져다 주라고 하겠습니다.

Mr. Kim: 감사합니다.

Nurse: 김선생님. 여기 심장약을 가지고 왔습니다. 지금 드셔도 됩니다.

Mr. Kim: 알겠습니다.

4. Blood Pressure (BP)
혈압

어휘퍼즐 정답

C	K	Y	N	P	D	I	H	N	I	U	E	L	W	X	T	A	F
J	V	I	K	M	I	X	W	Q	O	G	L	E	D	I	U	S	G
A	K	E	Q	A	A	C	J	S	Q	I	T	U	A	G	Y	I	O
K	V	N	I	J	S	M	T	P	O	V	K	X	R	S	Q	Q	S
L	U	K	G	N	T	B	T	Q	T	Q	S	Q	T	W	T	H	C
U	C	K	H	G	O	L	O	G	R	Q	Y	O	E	F	V	K	G
Y	J	B	H	A	L	O	C	W	W	L	L	X	R	N	B	J	B
Q	X	X	Y	Y	I	O	F	U	S	I	V	F	Y	F	F	C	J
B	L	S	P	K	C	D	B	X	C	X	W	P		D	N	X	A
R	K	O	E	T			X		I	U	I	X	W	T	E	H	Q
W	K	B	R	D	P	P	P	F	V	I	J	I	A	M	W	T	Y
K	K	B	T	T	R	R	T	H	J	U	N	C	L	E	G	A	P
H	B	B	E	R	E	E	R	N	C	R	S	B	L	E	N	V	Q
T	S	P	N	S	S	S	B	Y	Q	B	H	G	U	R	C	V	W
B	M	Q	S	P	S	S	N	H	C	Q	D	E	Y	H	O	C	T
T	P	U	I	Q	U	U	B	K	P	I	Q	A	B	M	K	J	F
F	R	U	O	A	R	R	K	E	O	N	X	N	G	N	X	P	I
E	D	X	N	K	E	E	A	U	K	G	O	J	M	O	I	G	H

Systolic pressure   Diastolic pressure   Blood pressure
Hypertension   Artery wall

독해구문

혈압이란?

간호사 또는 다른 의료진들이 혈압계와 청진기로 측정하는 혈압은 동맥벽에 가해지는 혈액의 압력입니다. 심장이 박동할 때마다, 심장은 동맥으로 피를 뿜어 보내고, 심장이 수축할 때 혈압은 최고치가 됩니다. 혈압을 잴 때 두 개의 수치가 기록됩니다. 더 높은 수치, 또는 수축기압은 심장이 수축하여 전신으로 혈액을 내뿜을 때 동맥 내벽에 가해지는 압력을 의미합니다. 더 낮은 수치, 또는 이완기압은 심장이 이완하고 혈액이 채워질 때 동맥내벽에 가해지는 압력을 의미합니다. 수축기압과 이완기압은 "mmHg"의 단위를 사용하여 기록됩니다. 이 수치는 수은 기둥이 혈압에 의하여 얼마나 높이 올라가는지를 표현합니다.

혈압계

펌프: 펌프는 몇 초 동안 당신의 동맥에서 혈류의 흐름을 막기 위해 커프를 부풀립니다.

다이얼: 숫자가 쓰여진 다이얼 또는 수은 기둥은 혈압수치를 기록하기 위해 사용됩니다.

밸브: 밸브는 혈류의 흐름을 재게할 수 있도록 커프에서 공기를 빠지도록 합니다.

커프: 커프는 상완에 감겨집니다.

혈압관련 주요구문

1. 혈압을 재기 전에 지켜야 할 주의사항이 있나요?
2. 체온과 혈압을 포함한 활력징후를 재겠습니다.
3. 혈압을 재겠습니다.
4. 전자동혈압계로 혈압을 재겠습니다.
5. 왼쪽 소매를 걷어 주시겠습니까?
6. 이 커프를 상완(팔뚝)에 감겠습니다.
7. 혈압수치를 재기 위해 커프에 공기를 주입할 것입니다.
8. 이 커프 안에 왼쪽 팔을 넣어주시겠습니까?
9. 커프가 부풀어질 때 압력을 상완(팔뚝)에서 느낄 것입니다.
10. 손에 일시적으로 감각이 무뎌지거나 저릿저릿함을 느낄 것입니다.
11. 청진기를 팔꿈치 안쪽의 접히는 부분에 대겠습니다.
12. 커프가 팔을 조인 후 서서히 느슨해질 것입니다.
13. 정상 혈압수치는 얼마인가요?
14. 제 나이에 적절한 혈압수치는 얼마인가요?
15. 내 혈압이 정상인가요?
16. 두 숫자는 무엇을 의미하지요?
17. 혈압은 120에 80입니다.

18. 혈압이 매우 높습니다.

19. 마지막으로 잰 혈압수치가 얼마인지 기억하나요?

20. 마지막으로 혈압을 잰 게 언제입니까?

혈압을 잴 때 유용한 정보

혈압 재기 30분 전에 커피를 마시거나 담배를 피우지 마세요.

검사하기 전에 화장실을 다녀오세요.

소변을 참으면 혈압수치가 변할 수 있습니다.

혈압을 재기 전에 등을 기대고 발은 땅에 대고 5분간 앉아계세요.

팔은 심장의 높이와 같게 검사 테이블에 올려 놓으세요.

혈압을 재는 동안 말하지 마세요.

나의 혈압 이야기

혈압계로 잰 혈압

Nurse: 요즘 건강상태가 어떻습니까?

Lorri: 어지럼증이 생겼어요.

Nurse: 알겠습니다. 고혈압이 있으십니까?

Lorri: 아니요. 고혈압증상이 전혀 없습니다.

Nurse: 보통 고혈압이 있는 분들은 증상이 거의 나타나지 않기 때문에 고혈압을 침묵의 살인자라고도 합니다. 혈압을 재겠습니다. 왼쪽 팔을 내미시고 소매를 걷어 주시겠습니까?

Lorri: 물론이죠.

Nurse: 자, 팔을 편안하게 하세요. 이 커프를 상완(팔뚝)에 감겠습니다. 조금 조일 것입니다. 그리고 커프가 부풀어질 때 손에 일시적으로 감각이 무뎌지거나 저릿저릿한 감각을 느끼실 것입니다.

Lorri: 알겠습니다.

Nurse: 이제 청진기를 팔꿈치 안쪽의 접히는 부분에 대겠습니다.

1분 후

Nurse: 끝났습니다. 혈압은 120/80입니다. 정상입니다.

Lorri: 두 숫자는 무엇을 의미하지요?

Nurse: 위의 숫자는 수축기압을 말합니다. 심장이 피를 심장 밖으로 뿜어낼 때 발생하는 압력입니다. 아래의 숫자는 확장기압입니다. 심장으로 혈액이 유입될 때 발생하는 압력입니다.

Lorri: 설명해 주셔서 감사합니다.

Nurse: 천만에요.

나의 혈압 이야기

전자동혈압계로 혈압 재기

Nurse: 어디 불편하신 곳이 있습니까?

Emily: 전혀 없습니다.

Nurse: 고혈압증상이 있었던 적이 있습니까?

Emily: 아니요. 제가 고혈압이 있던 적은 없습니다.

Nurse: 알겠습니다. 이제, 전자동혈압계로 혈압을 재겠습니다. 혈압수치를 알 수 있습니다.

Emily: 알겠습니다.

Nurse: 우선, 지시사항을 알려드리겠습니다. 먼저 왼쪽 소매를 걷어주세요. 그리고 커프 안에 왼쪽 팔을 넣어주세요. 커프가 팔을 조인 후 서서히 느슨해질 것입니다.

Emily: 알겠습니다.

Nurse: 편안히 있으세요.

1 분 후

Nurse: 다 끝났습니다. 혈압은 150/100입니다.

Emily: 음, 혈압수치가 너무 높게 나온 것 같아서 그러는데 혹시 다시 잴 수 있을까요?

Nurse: 물론이지요. 5분 후에 다시 재시면 됩니다. 그리고, 사람의 혈압은 하루 24시간 동안 변할 수 있습니다.

Emily: 정말이요? 몰랐습니다. 알려주셔서 감사합니다.

5. Respiratory Rate (RR)

호흡수

어휘퍼즐정답

U	B	Q	D	O	M	I	R	K	J	G	G	J	M	V	G
Y	C	N	E	D	H	S	E	A	A	N	I	E	P	J	D
D	P	O	M	L	O	Q	S	U	X	Q	J	B	W	N	U
R	Y	Q	X	R	S	J	P	I	Y	A	X	E	A	M	P
B	G	C	I	K	F	U	I	D	F	P	M	O	P	P	L
J	N	M	S	C	U	A	R	O	H	N	I	D	P	G	U
W	J	B	T	X	B	U	A	J	Y	E	T	F	W	T	F
U	V	M	W	H	H	I	T	Y	A	A	P	D	G	E	S
Q	V	J	G	T	S	M	O	I	C	Q	N	C	V	A	H
T	F	L	X	L	L	H	R	H	U	F	X	E	X	E	T
M	M	Y	L	D	T	E	Y	R	S	W	M	G	W	H	H
W	G	Y	C	Y	L	P		W	E	R	I	T	F	S	P
L	K	P	G	O	N	N	R	L	O	Q	F	E	I	G	G
O	C	Q	L	E	W	D	A	K	K	K	I	J	X	N	Y
P	F	B	A	F	Q	V	T	H	E	I	U	Q	H	K	U
B	R	A	D	Y	P	N	E	A	U	I	V	I	H	D	D

respiratory rate bradypnea apnea
tachypnea

독해구문

호흡수란?

호흡수 또는 호흡률은 편안한 상태의 일분 동안 내쉬는 호흡수입니다. 호흡수는 환자의 흉부가 오르고 내리는 수를 세어 잴 수 있습니다. 개인의 정상호흡률은 나이에 따라 변할 수 있습니다. 그리고 비정상적으로 빠르거나 느린 호흡은 특정 질환을 암시할 수 있습니다. 호흡이 정상인지, 비정상적으로 빠른지, 느린지 또는 무호흡증인지를 발견하는 것이 목적입니다.

나의 호흡수 이야기

나의 활력징후

Nurse: 오늘 어떠십니까? 제가 담당간호사입니다.

Patient: 아주 좋습니다. 감사합니다.

Nurse: 몇 가지 확인하겠습니다. 이름과 생년월일을 말씀해주세요.

Patient: 제프리 존슨이고 1976년 11월 06일 생입니다.

Nurse: 감사합니다. 존슨선생님, 몸무게와 키를 먼저 재고 활력징후를 재겠습니다.

Mr. Johnson: 알겠습니다.

Nurse: 키와 몸무게를 재기 위해 신장계가 부착된 저울을 사용합니다.

Mr. Johnson: 신장계가 무엇인가요?

Nurse: 신장계는 환자의 머리 위에서 멈춰서는 측정막대가 부착되어있는 세로로 된 자 입니다. 신발을 벗고 여기 저울발판에 올라서세요.

Mr. Johnson: 알겠습니다.

Nurse: 뒷꿈치, 엉덩이와 견갑골(어깨뼈)이 측정대에 닿아야 합니다. 또한, 앞을 똑바로 보고, 가능한 한 키를 곧추세우고 숨을 들이 쉬세요. 자세를 확인하겠습니다.

Mr. Johnson: 제가 자세를 제대로 했나요?

Nurse: 예. 측정막대가 내려와서 환자의 정수리부분에 닿을 겁니다. 그리고 키와 몸무게를 기록할 겁니다.

몇 초 후

Nurse: 저울에서 내려오셔서 신발을 신으세요. 몸무게는 70킬로그램이고 키는 182센티미터입니다.

Mr. Johnson: 알겠습니다.

Nurse: 이제 활력징후를 측정하겠습니다. 이 의자에 앉아주세요.

Mr. Johnson: 여기요?

Nurse: 예. 체온을 먼저 재겠습니다. 이쪽을 보세요. 36.7°C입니다. 이제 맥박을 재겠습니다. 팔을 주시겠습니까?

Mr. Johnson: 여기요.

1 분 후

Nurse: 맥박은 80이고 호흡수는 17입니다. 지금까지의 결과들이 아주 좋습니다.

Mr. Johnson: 제 호흡수도 잰 줄 몰랐습니다.

Nurse: 제가 맥박을 잴 때 호흡수도 쟀습니다.

Mr. Johnson: 호흡수는 어떻게 재나요?

Nurse: 음. 환자의 흉부를 보며 1분 정도 호흡수를 셉니다. 그러나, 만일 환자가 정상적으로 호흡을 하다면 약 30초 정도 잰 환자의 호흡수에 곱하기 2를 합니다.

Mr. Johnson: 알겠습니다. 설명해주셔서 감사합니다.

Nurse: 천만에요. 혈압을 재겠습니다. 소매를 걷어 주세요.

1 분 후

Nurse: 혈압은 90에 60입니다.

Mr. Johnson: 너무 낮은 가요?

Nurse: 정상범위에 있습니다. 어지러웠던 적이 있었나요?

Mr. Johnson: 아니요.

Nurse: 그렇다면 걱정 안하셔도 됩니다. 낮은 혈압이 높은 혈압보다 훨씬 더 나아요.

References:

www.chp.edu

"Needle Phobia", 2007, Jerry Emanualson, NeedlePhobia.com

"Needle Phobia: The Neglected Diagnosis", 1995, James G. Hamilton, M.D., Journal of Family Practice

"Needle Phobia Information", Date Unknown, D. Keith Lamb, The Needle Phobia Information Site http://www.healthcentral.com/anxiety/disorder-types-273889-5.html

www.cholesterollevelschart.net

wiki.answers.com

www. hcrefund.com

www.goodhormonehealth.com

www. dentonregional.com

www.jewishhospitalcincinnati.com

guides.machinescience.org

Saunders Comprehensive Review for the NCLEX-RN Examination, 3rd edition, by Linda Anne Silvestri Reference: Expert 10-Minute Physical Examinations, 1997, Mosby's

www.albireo

www.ama-assn.org

www.yalemedicalgroup.org

www.buzzle.com

www.wisc-online.com

www.sthelenahospitals.org

www. nhlbi.nih.gov

www. edb.utexas.edu

www.wisegeek.com

www.wisc-online.com

www.knowledgebase-script.com